CORONARY CINEMATOGRAPHY

CORONARY CINEMATOGRAPHY

CURTIS E. GREEN, M.D.

Professor of Radiology and Medicine (Cardiology)
Georgetown University School of Medicine
Director, Cardiac Radiology
Georgetown University Medical Center
Washington, District of Columbia

LIPPINCOTT–RAVEN PUBLISHERS

PHILADELPHIA

ACQUISITIONS EDITOR: JAMES D. RYAN
PROJECT EDITOR: MOLLY E. DICKMEYER
PRODUCTION MANAGER: CAREN ERLICHMAN
PRODUCTION COORDINATOR: DAVID YURKOVICH
DESIGN COORDINATOR: KATHY KELLEY-LUEDTKE
INDEXER: LYNNE E. MAHAN
COMPOSITOR: REED TECHNOLOGY
PRINTER: QUEBECOR/KINGSPORT

Library of Congress Cataloging-in-Publication Data

Green, Curtis E.
     Coronary cinematography / Curtis E. Green.
         p.   cm.
     Includes bibliographical references and index.
     ISBN (invalid) 0-397-51300-1 (alk. paper)
     1. Cineangiography. 2. Coronary heart disease—Imaging.
I.   Title.
     [DNLM: 1. Coronary Vessels—anatomy & histology.   2. Coronary Angiography.   3. Coronary Disease—pathology.   4. Cineangiography. WG 500   G795c   1996]
RC683.5.C54G74   1996
616.1'2307572—dc20
DNLM/DLC
for Library of Congress   95-152
                                                                    CIP

The material contained in this volume was submitted as previously unpublished material, except in the instances in which credit has been given to the source from which some of the illustrative material was derived.

Great care has been taken to maintain the accuracy of the information contained in the volume. However, neither Lippincott–Raven Publishers nor the editors can be held responsible for errors or for any consequences arising from the use of the information herein. The authors and publisher have exerted every effort to ensure that drug selection and dosage set forth in this text are in accord with current recommendations and practice at the time of publication. However, in view of ongoing research, changes in government regulation, and the constant flow of information relating to drug therapy and drug reactions, the reader is urged to check the package insert for each drug for any change in indications and dosage and for added warnings and precautions. This is particularly important when the recommended agent is a new or infrequently employed drug.

Materials appearing in this book prepared by individuals as part of their official duties as U.S. Government employees are not covered by the above-mentioned copyright.

9   8   7   6   5   4   3   2   1

This book is dedicated to my wife, Lisa,
and daughter Clare, and to the memory
of Edward E. Christensen, M.D.,
friend, mentor, and radiologist
extraordinaire.

PREFACE

The impetus for writing this book was the persistent inquiries by the cardiology fellows about where they could read about the things we discussed around the cine projector as we reviewed the day's coronary angiograms. Although there are a myriad of excellent texts about coronary anatomy and physiology, coronary artery disease, and the technical skills involved in cannulating the coronary arteries, little has been written about how to ensure that the end result — the coronary angiogram — is as high quality as possible. When all is said and done, what coronary angiography is really about is taking pictures, and in reality, the angiographer is a medical cinematographer. That the study must be performed in as safe a manner as possible goes without saying, but a safe angiogram that yields inadequate or incorrect information is worse than no angiogram at all. Unfortunately, many angiographers seem to know far more about taking pictures safely than about making sure that the pictures are of excellent quality.

What I have tried to do in this text is recreate those sessions around the projector. This has proven to be a difficult task, and I am certain that as these words go to press I will have already thought of dozens of things I could have explained better or should have added to the discussion. Nevertheless, I believe that the precepts and techniques discussed in these chapters can provide a sound foundation in coronary angiographic techniques for both the novice and the experienced coronary angiographer. For those of you in the former category, do not be discouraged or overwhelmed by the volume of information; it will all make sense as you acquire more experience and expertise. Those of you in the latter group may find some new information here or be reminded of things learned long ago but since forgotten.

The organization of this book is based on a stepwise progression through the areas of knowledge that I believe must be understood if one is to become an excellent coronary cinematographer. Chapter 1 deals with the universally dreaded subject of physics. It is not a compendium of formulas and information irrelevant to the average physician, but rather a brief discussion of topics that have a direct bearing on cineangiographic quality. Chapters 2 and 4 cover coronary artery anatomy and abnormalities, respectively. Except for the information on coronary anomalies, much of this information will be old hat to the experienced angiographer and is included primarily for the benefit of the neophyte. Chapter 3, on the other hand, contains information that I have never seen written down in one place and is the primary reason for the existence of this book. Chapter 3 contains a detailed discussion of not only the basics of axial coronary angiography but also the subtle points such as why a certain view helps in one patient and not in another and how to tailor each view to maximize its value. Chapter 5 is a discussion of measuring coronary stenoses. It describes the basic options and limitations of the techniques, as well as my personal philosophy. It is not intended, however, to be an exhaustive reference on quantitative coronary angiography. Chapter 6 serves as a wrap-up and deals with how one can use an understanding of physics, anatomy, and angiographic technique to ensure that the coronary angiogram is of as high quality as possible under the existing circumstances of equipment, patient, and anatomy.

It is my belief, based on personal experience teaching dozens of cardiology fellows to interpret coronary angiograms, that the information contained herein, when understood and properly applied, will result in the best chance of obtaining angiograms that minimize errors of both omission and commission. There is no doubt that trying to apply these principles requires significantly more mental work than a rote approach, but the rewards are well worth that price. Your patients deserve no less. One final word of advice: never assume that because you have seen a lot of angiograms that you have seen all possible variations. Even after reading over 15,000 coronary studies, I see new things every week. That is a part of what makes this job so interesting!

On a technical note, all of the illustrations in this text were prepared using a personal computer. Cineangiograms were digitized with a Nikon LS3510AF film scanner using Aldus Photostyler to adjust brightness and contrast. Images were imported as Tagged Image Format (TIF) files into Microsoft Powerpoint, where they were scaled, cropped, and labeled. They were then printed on a Mitsubishi sublimation dye color printer. I believe that this process has provided significantly better image quality and uniformity than is available with conventional photographic techniques at a considerably lower cost.

ACKNOWLEDGMENTS

There are many people whose efforts throughout the years have indirectly contributed to this effort, and I would like to recognize a few who were particularly important to me. In addition to trying to teach me to be a good radiologist, my mentors during radiology residency at Parkland Hospital instilled in me a love of understanding why things look like they do and of teaching. For this I am particularly grateful to Jack Reynolds, who gave me my first opportunities to teach, Michael Landay, Tom Curry, George Curry, and the late Ed Christensen. My friend John Moore deserves a special thanks for my early education in the whys and wherefores of radiographic equipment. It was George Curry who first got me interested in cardiac radiology and then helped me obtain my fellowship at the University of California at San Diego, where I had the good fortune to learn from two outstanding cardiac radiologists, Michael Kelley and Charles Higgins. Mike Kelley, in turn, was in large part responsible for my first real job, staff radiologist at the University of Alabama at Birmingham, and has continued over the years to be a friend and advisor. At the University of Alabama at Birmingham, I began a career-long professional relationship with Larry Elliott, my division chief at Birmingham and chairman at Georgetown University. Over the years, Dr. Elliott has been an invaluable source of knowledge and advice and has provided me with both the tools and opportunity to learn the trade of cardiac radiology. I am grateful for his ongoing support. Without it this book would not have been possible. Early during my career I also had the good fortune to become acquainted with William Barnett of Cinerex who, along with his colleagues, taught me at least half of what I know about x-ray and film techinque.

By necessity, a larger part of my career has been spent in the company of cardiologists than in that of radiologists. I am fortunate to have worked closely with a number of excellent angiographers with whom I could learn and trade ideas. When I first started at Georgetown, there was no history of cardiac radiology in the catheterization laboratory, but Al Del Negro, the director of the laboratories, accepted me without hesitation and helped create a beneficial working environment. With out his help, I could never have established myself. That tradition was continued by Kenneth Kent and Stephen Oesterle during each of their tenures as catheterization laboratory director and allowed me to work in a friendly and supportive environment where I could learn, teach, and mature as a specialist in cardiac diseases. Especially strong support came from one of my former fellows at the University of Alabama at Birmingham, Lowell Satler, who joined the faculty at Georgetown after completion of his training. Lowell's support and friendship have been critical to my career development. Although far too numerous to mention individually, the support and friendship many of the other cardiologists, both at the University of Alabama at Birmingham and Georgetown, has also been appreciated. It also has been my pleasure to teach and learn from an outstanding group of cardiology fellows over the years and to serve for a time as their fellowship director. I know of no other radiologist who has had that privilege. Their friendship, support, and respect have made my job a pleasure.

A number of people deserve special recognition for their more direct role in this project. I would especially like to thank William Oetgen, Julie Kovach, and Jonathan Safren for reviewing the manuscript. Their suggestions proved immensely helpful. William Davros was a valuable resource for both the text and illustrations in the physics chapter. I am also indebted to Jeffrey Popma for assistance and encouragement in using digital reproduction of the illustrations, to Moshe Mehlman for production of the prints, and to Harold Benson and Cate Bozarth for helping me obtain the equipment that made this possible. Without their help I would probably still be laboriously hand-labeling illustration.

Lastly, thanks to my colleagues in radiology for covering for me while I typed away, and to my wife, Lisa, for putting up with my frantic efforts to finish this text only a few months late.

CONTENTS

CORONARY CINEMATOGRAPHY

Coronary Cinematography, by Curtis E. Green.
Lippincott–Raven Publishers, © 1995.

CHAPTER ONE

Basic Imaging Physics

All modern cineangiography systems are microprocessor controlled; for the most part, they operate in an automatic fashion, requiring a minimum of operator input. As a result, catheterization laboratory personnel tend to forget that these systems require a fair amount of preventative maintenance and some attention to detail if they are to reliably produce high quality cineangiograms. Fortunately, there are some relatively simple steps that can be taken to ensure that cine systems function in a reliable fashion and that the quality of the angiograms is optimal. It is the purpose of this chapter to convey a basic knowledge of how a cine system works, so that the reader will be better able to recognize when problems arise and know where to look for help in resolving them. A basic understanding of imaging physics is an essential part of the expertise required to perform high quality cineangiography.

X-RAYS

X-rays are a form of electromagnetic radiation and are related to such common forms of energy as radio and television waves, infrared and ultraviolet light, visible light, and gamma rays. These various types of electromagnetic radiation differ in their wave lengths, which vary from 10^{-14} m for gamma rays to 3000 m for some radio waves. Most diagnostic x-rays have wavelengths between 10^{-10} and 10^{-11} m. In addition to behaving like waves, x-rays also have some of the properties of particles. Because of this feature, an x-ray beam can be thought of as consisting of individual packets of energy, referred to as photons.

1

COMPONENTS OF A CINEANGIOGRAPHY SYSTEM

Regardless of manufacturer or design, all modern catheterization laboratory systems have certain elements in common. They basically consist of an x-ray tube with collimators, a gantry to support the x-ray tube and imaging system, a table to support the patient, an image intensifier with optical distributor, imaging devices (television and cine cameras), a film processor, and a projector (Fig. 1-1). The quality of the image depends on the proper functioning of each of these elements.

X-Ray Tube

X-rays are produced from the conversion of energy that occurs when a stream of electrons collides with the tungsten target of an x-ray tube. This is a very inefficient process and results in conversion of approximately 1% of the energy of the electron beam into x-rays and the remainder into heat. It is this high heat production that largely limits x-ray tube output and partly determines cine quality.

The primary elements of an x-ray tube are the anode (positively charged), the cathode with its tungsten filament (negatively charged), the focusing cup, and the target. These elements are surrounded by an evacuated glass envelope (Fig. 1-2). Current flowing through the tungsten filament generates heat, which causes electrons to move away from the surface of the filament. The electrons are accelerated across the vacuum by the positive charge on the anode. They strike the target, which is made of a carbon disc coated with a tungsten-rhenium alloy. A charge on the focusing cup ensures that the electrons strike only a small area of the target, the focal spot. The x-rays produced by this interaction are emitted in all directions; the heat generated is conducted away from the target by the anode.

To prevent the overheating that would result from constant bombardment of one area of the target, the anode rotates at a high number of revolutions per minute so that a new area is constantly presented to the electron beam. Part of the delay that occurs at the beginning of each cine exposure is a result of the time required to accelerate the anode. (The anode rotates more slowly during fluoroscopy or when no x-rays are being produced than it does during cine runs.)

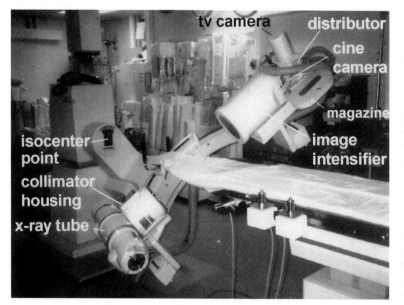

Figure 1-1. Cardiac catheterization laboratory. The gantry is positioned for a caudal left anterior oblique view. Because neither the patient nor the table need be moved to obtain longitudinal (caudal or cranial) angulation, the amount of angulation is independent of the amount of rotation in the transverse plane. The pivot point for the C-arm determines the isocenter point regardless of the amount of displacement of the image intensifier away from the table.

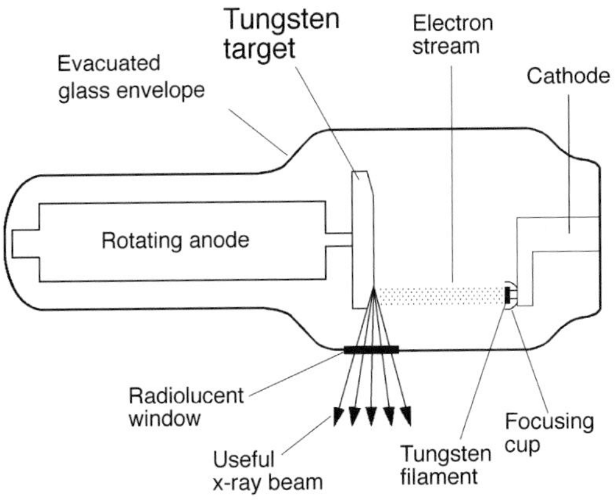

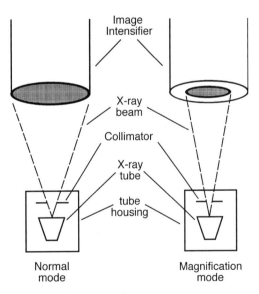

Figure 1-2. Diagram of a rotating anode x-ray tube.

Collimators

To minimize patient exposure, the size of the x-ray beam must be restricted to conform to the size of the image intensifier during fluoroscopy, or to the size of the cine film during cine filming. This is accomplished by movable lead sheets called collimators. Because image intensifiers are round, the first level of collimation is achieved by an iris-like collimator. The aperture of this collimator automatically changes each time the magnification mode changes (Fig. 1-4), so that the patient is not irradiated outside the area of imaging.

A second level of collimation is necessary during cine filming because the film is rectangular and the image intensifier is round. Either part of the film or part of the radiation must be wasted. The relation between the amount of film exposed and the proportion of the image intensifier used is referred to as the cine framing, and it has an effect on the size of the image seen on film (Fig. 1-5). The most frequently used

A second method for reducing the heat burden of the target is to angle the target so that the apparent focal spot is smaller than the actual focal spot (Fig. 1-3). The target angle is typically about 11 degrees. All of the heat is then dissipated through the glass envelope, which is cooled by air, oil, or both.

Because the x-rays are emitted in all directions, the housing for the x-ray tube is lined with lead; only a small area is left for emission of x-rays. Government regulations require that the tube shielding must allow no more than 100 mR of radiation to leak from the tube in 1 hour of operation at maximum continuous rated power.

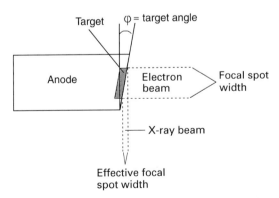

Figure 1-3. Because the target is angled relative to the electron beam, the apparent or effective focal spot is smaller than the actual focal spot. This allows greater tube heating with no loss of resolution.

Figure 1-4. Diagram of the relation between the automatic collimator and the image intensifier mode. The collimator is wide open when the entire intensifier is used for imaging *(left)* and closes to adjust to the smaller imaging area in magnification mode *(right)*.

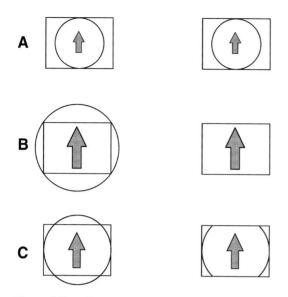

Figure 1-5. Effect of cine framing on image size. The rectangles correspond to the shape of the cine film and the circles to the shape of the image intensifier output. **(A)** Exact framing, or underframing, results in the smallest film image, but all of the image intensifier output is used. **(B)** Total overframing results in the largest film image, but a significant portion of the image intensifier output is unused. **(C)** Maximum horizontal framing results in a reasonable compromise between image size and use of intensifier output. Collimation of the intensifier output to the cine framing is mandatory in all but underframing, in which all of the image intensifier output is used.

method of cine framing is *maximum horizontal overframing*, which provides a good compromise between the shape of the cine film and that of the radiation field. Because part of the x-ray field is not used for imaging, collimators must be used to block off the unused radiation. This is usually accomplished with a rectangular collimator, although one manufacturer uses an octagonal collimator. These collimators can work either automatically or manually. The manual varieties allow the operator to "cone down" to within cine framing but can result in overexposure of the patient if they are left outside the portion of the image intensifier that is seen by the cine film.

Grid

A certain number of x-rays interact with tissue by being scattered rather than absorbed (see Interaction of X-Rays With Tissue). Because their direction of travel after leaving the body is random, these scattered x-rays do not carry any diagnostic information but may strike the image intensifier and expose the film. There are several ways to decrease scatter. One of the most effective is the x-ray grid, a flat plate composed of thin lead strips alternating with strips of a radiolucent material, which is placed against the face of the image intensifier. The lead strips stop scattered x-ray photons that are not traveling in a relatively straight direction, and the radiolucent strips allow nonscattered x-rays through to the image intensifier (Fig. 1-6). Film quality is substantially enhanced by using a grid, and all modern systems do so; however, because some of the x-rays do not reach the intensifier when a

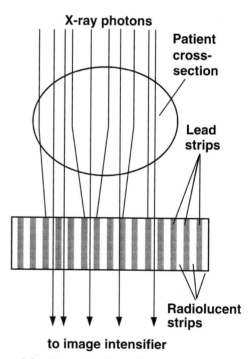

Figure 1-6. Diagram of a radiographic grid. Lead strips absorb most of the scattered photons (and some of the nonscattered ones).

grid is used, exposure must be increased to maintain image brightness. The overall benefit is well worth this price.

Image Intensifier

The image intensifier (Fig. 1-7) converts x-rays into light and allows a substantially lower x-ray dose to be used than would otherwise be required. X-ray photons exiting the patient strike the input phosphor, an aluminum plate coated with cesium iodide crystals, which converts the x-ray energy into blue light. The light then strikes an antimony photocathode and is converted into electrons. The electrons are accelerated across the intensifier by a potential of about 30,000 V and are focused to strike the zinc cadmium output phosphor, which converts them into green light. This green light is readily detected by the eye as well as by a television camera or photographic film.

One of the advantages of the image intensifier is its ability to increase the brightness of the image. This is accomplished by two mechanisms, minification and acceleration of electrons across the intensifier. Minification brightness gain results from the "shrinking" of the image as it travels from the input to the output phosphors. Light collected over the large area of the input phosphor is focused on the much smaller area of the output phosphor, resulting in a considerable gain in brightness. In addition, the high potential of the intensifier causes the electrons to strike the output phosphor with more energy, resulting in more light output. The combination of these two factors results in a substantial brightness gain, allowing a significant reduction in x-ray dose. There is a lower limit of dose, however, below which there is an insufficient number of x-ray photons to allow accurate definition of the vessel. This is determined in large part by the size of the object being imaged and is ultimately independent of the sophistication of the x-ray system.

Most modern catheterization laboratories use multimode image intensifiers so that the amount of magnification can be varied depending on the application. Although some radiology laboratories use image intensifiers as large as 17 inches (43 cm), cardiac laboratories usually have intensifiers with a maximum field size of 9 inches (23 cm). The degree of magnification is determined by the percentage of the intensifier face that is used for imaging, and this is controlled by electronic focusing (Fig. 1-8). In low magnification mode (e.g., 9-inch mode), the entire intensifier face is used. In higher magnification modes, only a portion of the intensifier face is used: two thirds of the diameter in 6-in (15-cm)

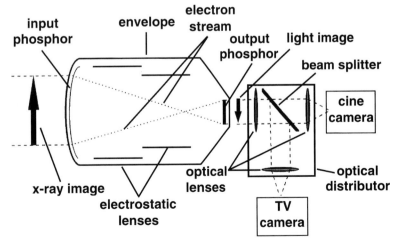

Figure 1-7. Diagram of an image intensifier and optic distributor. The x-ray image is converted to an electron stream by the input phosphor, then focused by the electrostatic lenses onto the output phosphor. The minified and brighter optical image generated by the output phosphor can then be directed to the television camera, cine camera, or other device by the optical distributor.

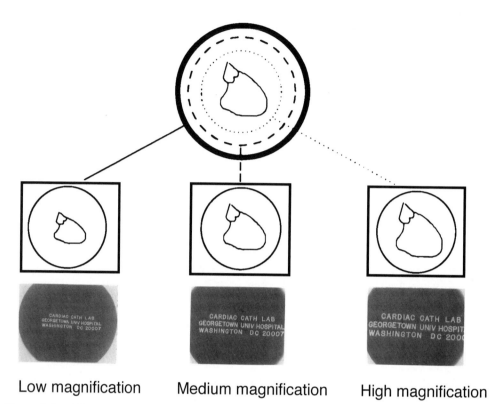

Low magnification   Medium magnification   High magnification

Figure 1-8. Effect of image intensifier mode on magnification. The image is progressively magnified as the field of view decreases (less of the intensifier face is used).

mode, half the diameter in 4.5-in (11.5-cm) mode. Magnification thus results because there is less minification in the higher magnification modes than in low magnification mode.

There is a secondary and undesirable effect of increasing magnification, however. Because there is less minification, there is also less minification brightness gain. At lowest magnification (9-inch mode in most systems), light is collected from an area of approximately 64 square inches (160 cm^2). This area is reduced to 3 square inches (8 cm^2) at the output phosphor, resulting in a brightness gain from minification of about 21. When 6-inch mode is used, the input area is only 28 square inches (71 cm^2), resulting in a gain of about 9, less than half of that produced in 9-inch mode. This decrease in minification brightness gain requires a proportionate increase in x-ray dose if film exposure is to remain constant. The same thing happens with a change

from 6-inch mode to 4.5-inch mode, which has a minification brightness gain of about 5. As a general rule, x-ray exposure must be approximately doubled with each stepped increase in magnification mode. This not only increases the exposure of the patient, but also increases the radiation exposure of the laboratory personnel and the workload of the equipment.

Optical Distributor

Light produced by the output phosphor of the image intensifier can be used to produce a television image or to expose x-ray film. The optical distributor is a device composed of a series of lenses and a mirror which directs and splits light according to the type of imaging desired (see Fig. 1-7). During fluoroscopy, all of the output of the intensifier is directed to the television camera, which requires a relatively small amount of light. X-ray film exposure requires considerably more light, so during cine filming the dose must be increased. During cine filming, approximately 85% of the light is sent to the cine camera; the remaining 15% is sent to the television camera to allow real-time monitoring of the cine run. Because more light goes to the film, less noise is produced on the film than on the television image. One manufacturer uses a 50-50 split between television and film to allow for better digital imaging, at the price of a slightly degraded film image.

Television Camera

A television camera converts light into an electronic signal by scanning a photoconductor, usually made of lead oxide, that has been exposed to the output of the image intensifier. This is done by passing an electron beam across the face of the photoconductor, generating a signal proportionate to the amount of light striking the photoconductor in each location. In the past, most systems used 525 scan lines, similar to the number used for a standard home television system. Currently, most cameras use more than 1000 scan lines; the exact number depends on the manufacturer. The former is referred to as low resolution television and the latter as high resolution television, although future systems may make 1000 lines look like low resolution.

There are two methods of scanning. The oldest and most commonly used method is *interlaced scanning*. In this method, the face of the output phosphor is scanned as a series of alternating lines, even-numbered lines on one pass and odd-numbered lines on the next. Each pass requires one-sixtieth of a second, so the entire image is scanned every one-thirtieth of a second. Persistence of the image on the television screen decreases the perception of flicker, which is normally visible with rates slower than 50 frames per second. Interlaced scanning requires continuous fluoroscopy. With a more recent method, *progressive scanning*, all lines are scanned sequentially in one-thirtieth of a sec-

ond. This method is commonly used with digital fluoroscopy and can be combined with pulsed fluoroscopy to reduce the radiation dose. Although some television systems can handle both types of scanning, the systems usually are not directly compatible. With either method, the final output to the television screen is usually interlaced to decrease flicker. (For a good example of flicker, notice that during cine filming at 30 frames per second, the fluoroscopic image seems to pulsate, whereas fluoroscopy provides a much smoother image.)

Cine Camera

In most laboratories, the final result is a cinematographic image recorded at 30 to 60 frames per second on 35-mm film. The cine camera consists of a lens, a film advance mechanism, a shutter, and a film magazine (see Fig. 1-1). The lens focuses the image formed on the output phosphor of the intensifier onto the film. The advance mechanism uses a claw to move the film between exposures; a rotating shutter cuts off light while the film is advanced.

The aperture of the cine camera lens is usually left wide open to decrease vignetting, the diminution in light intensity at the edge of the field. Adjustments in light input to the camera can be readily made by placing an aperture in front of the objective lens of the camera. Although ready-made apertures are available, a piece of exposed x-ray film with a hole cut in the center serves equally well. The size of the hole is determined by examination of the density and sensitometry strips (see Chap. 6) and calculation of the increase or decrease in light necessary to achieve an average density of about 0.85 optical units. In systems that use an electronic aperture, adjustments must be made by the service personnel.

Gantry

Advances in x-ray gantry design have made possible all of the angulated views that are necessary for coronary angiography. Several designs by various suppliers are currently used to achieve compound angulations, and all of these designs work relatively well. In some of the older designs (e.g., Siemens Cardioskop-U, Philips Cardiodiagnost-C, General Electric LU-C), the amount of cranial or caudal angulation depended on the amount of tube rotation in the transverse plane. In more recent systems by all manufacturers, this is no longer true. Most manufacturers claim cranial and caudal limits of 45 degrees. Unfortunately, these limits can rarely be achieved with a patient on the table unless isocenter is ignored (see Chap. 3).

PRODUCTION OF X-RAYS

The output of the x-ray tube during any given exposure is determined by three factors: the tube current, the tube voltage, and the exposure time. *Tube current* is the flow of electrons from the cathode to the anode. This is measured in milliamperes (mA) and is proportional to the number of x-ray photons produced. The *energy of the x-ray beam* is determined by the potential (voltage) across the x-ray tube between the cathode and the anode and is measured in thousands of electron volts (keV). Because x-ray beams are not monochromatic (i.e., not all photons have the same energy), peak kilovoltage of the beam (kVp) is used as an indicator of beam energy. The average kilovoltage is one third to one half of the kVp. X-ray photons of insufficient energy to pass through the patient are removed from the x-ray beam by an aluminum filter placed between the x-ray source and the patient. The *exposure time*, or *pulse width*, is the time during which the x-ray beam is produced. During continuous fluoroscopy, this can run from seconds to minutes; cine exposure times are usually between 2.5 and 10 msec per exposure.

Because the x-ray beam is ultimately converted to light by the image intensifier, the situation is somewhat analogous to that encountered with everyday photography. The kVp cor-

responds to the type of light used for imaging in a camera, usually the visible spectrum, but occasionally, infrared. The tube current and pulse width correspond to aperture (f-stop) and shutter speed, respectively. In a camera, the desired exposure can be maintained by varying the f-stop and shutter speed inversely. In an x-ray system, there is a similar interplay between exposure time and tube current. For a given kVp, proper exposure of the x-ray film is determined by the product of the tube current in milliamperes (mA) and the pulse width in seconds (s); the product is measured in milliampere-seconds and is abbreviated mAs. If tube current is doubled, the pulse width can be halved, and vice versa. In cine systems, the kVp does not remain fixed, which adds another variable to the equation. As discussed elsewhere in this chapter, kVp has significant effects on image quality, film density, radiation dose to personnel in the laboratory, and equipment workload.

The ability of an x-ray tube to absorb and dissipate heat is a major factor in how well the tube performs. With a constant potential generator such as those used for cinefluorography, the amount of heat generated by a single exposure, expressed in heat units (HU), is proportional to the product of the kVp, the tube current, and the pulse width.

$$HU = 1.4(kVp \times mAs)$$

Manufacturers usually express tube heat tolerance in terms of the heat storage capacity of the housing. Depending on the model, this can vary from 375,000 to 1,500,000 HU. This is significantly more than the anode can tolerate, so the housing must be able to draw heat away from the anode assembly in an efficient fashion.

Another important factor is the *kilowatt rating* of an x-ray tube, which is operationally defined as the ability of the x-ray tube to make a single exposure of 100 msec. It is equal to the product of the kVp and the tube current. A 100-kW tube is one that is able to sustain a 100-msec exposure of 100 kVp and 1000 mA.

$$100 \text{ kVp} \times 1000 \text{ mA} = 100,000 \text{ W, or } 100 \text{ kW}$$

The kilowatt rating of an x-ray tube is dependent on many factors, but for our purposes, the most important is focal spot size. As previously described, the focal spot is the area of the target that is bombarded by the electron beam. Smaller focal spots tolerate less heat loading but, within limits, allow better resolution. Because most x-ray tubes have two focal spots, the kilowatt rating is expressed as two numbers. For example, a 35/100-kW tube has a kilowatt rating of 35 kW on the small focal spot and 100 kW on the large focal spot. Effective focal spot sizes vary among models but are usually 0.3 to 0.6 mm for small and 0.8 to 1.2 mm for large focal spots. These are nominal sizes; the actual focal spot size may be as much as 50% greater (see Fig. 1-3).

CONTROL OF X-RAY EXPOSURE

Because of the relatively small radiographic field of the image intensifier, it is frequently impossible to fit the entire heart into the field of view. This necessitates moving the patient *(panning)*, which in turn requires that the x-ray exposure be modified as the cine run progresses so that proper film density is maintained. Because this requires millisecond-to-millisecond variation in x-ray factors, control is maintained by a microprocessor in the cine generator. The goal in establishing exposure factors is to provide the lowest kVp consistent with penetration of the patient by a sufficient number of photons and the highest mAs allowed by tube heating constraints. Factors taken into consideration by the generator include frame rate, pulse width, maximum cine run duration, focal spot size, tube heating, and tube heat storage capacity. Given these parameters, the generator makes a series of test exposures and sets the kVp and the tube current to give the desired exposure. The factors vary with patient size and angiographic view; for example, caudally angled views require higher factors than nonangled views (see Chap. 3).

As described previously, tube heating is a prime limiting factor in how well the x-ray tube performs and thus directly affects the quality of the angiogram. Increasing the kVp is a more efficient way to increase film density than is increasing the mAs, and it also results in less tube heating. In the usual range of diagnostic x-ray energies, the same change in film density can be obtained with an increase of 10 kVp as with a doubling of the mAs, but at a substantially lower heat load. From a practical standpoint, this means that the generator has more leeway in making changes in kVp than in tube current. Although efficient, increasing the kVp has the disadvantage of degrading image quality. Another means of adjusting exposure is to allow the pulse width to change while keeping the tube current and kVp constant until the preset pulse width limit is exceeded. A third technique, electronically changing the iris of the cine camera, has the disadvantage of decreasing dose and thus increasing noise as aperture size is increased, but it allows for a larger range of exposure over which kVp can be kept in an optimal range.

INTERACTION OF X-RAYS WITH TISSUE

X-ray images are capable of providing anatomic detail because x-rays interact differently with various parts of the body. For our purposes, there are two main types of tissue interaction that affect the quality of the radiographic image. *Compton scattering* occurs when an x-ray photon collides with an outer-shell electron of an atom. In the collision, part of the energy of the photon is given to the electron, so that the photon exits the atom in a different direction from that at which it entered and with a lower energy (Fig. 1-9). If the photon then leaves the body and strikes the image intensifier, it will create an image that is not a true representation of the anatomic part being imaged. This phenomenon is referred to as scatter.

A second interaction, the *photoelectric effect*, occurs when an x-ray photon collides with an inner-shell electron and is completely absorbed

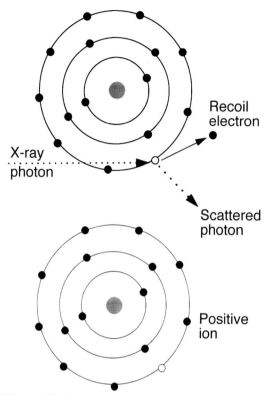

the material through which it passes. If there is a good match in energy between the x-ray beam and the k-edge of the atom, then the photoelectric effect will predominate. The k-edge is different for each element, but in general, the photoelectric effect is maximized at lower beam energies, and Compton scattering increases as the kVp increases. An excellent example of this phenomenon is the use of iodinated contrast material, for which x-ray absorption begins to drop off as the kVp rises above 75 or 80. Similarly, on a weight-for-weight basis, tin is a better absorber of x-rays than lead with energies up to 88 kVp, the k-edge of lead.

Figure 1-9. Compton scattering. The x-ray photon has been deflected by an outer-shell electron, producing a scattered photon, a recoil electron, and a positive ion. Depending on how much energy remains in the scattered photon, it may exit the patient and reach the image intensifier.

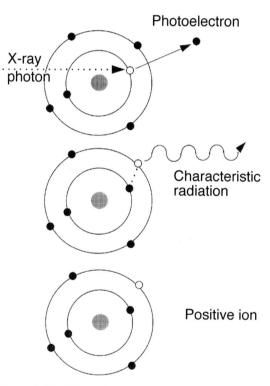

(Fig. 1-10). The electron is ejected from the atom, creating a vacancy that is filled by an outer-shell electron. This process creates a secondary x-ray photon (i.e., characteristic radiation) which is frequently of low enough energy to be completely absorbed by the body or by the filter of the x-ray tube. This is desirable from an imaging standpoint, because each photon in the original beam is either absorbed through the photoelectric effect or passes straight through to strike the image intensifier.

The ratio of x-rays absorbed through the photoelectric effect compared with those deflected by Compton scattering depends on the energy of the x-ray beam and the composition of

Figure 1-10. Photoelectric effect. If the energy of the x-ray photon is similar to that of an inner-shell electron, the photon is absorbed. The characteristic radiation that results as an outer-shell electron drops down to replace the dislodged inner-shell electron is usually absorbed by the body of the patient and does not reach the image intensifier.

FACTORS AFFECTING IMAGE QUALITY

The overall quality of a radiographic image is a function of two main parameters, contrast and resolution, each of which is affected by numerous factors. Contrast is the difference in density between various areas on the radiograph. The term resolution refers to the ability of the image to discern small differences in geometry (spatial resolution) or in contrast (contrast resolution). Contrast and resolution are closely related.

Contrast

Contrast is a function of both the inherent properties of the object being imaged (subject contrast) and certain technical factors. Subject contrast is affected by differences in thickness and composition of the object or objects (i.e.,

the heart and coronary arteries) and can be altered by the addition of contrast material. Less obvious are the profound effects that both angiographic and radiographic technique can have on contrast (Fig. 1-11). Of major importance is the use of the lowest practical kVp. As discussed previously, this has two salutary effects: enhanced absorption of x-rays by iodinated contrast material and increased photoelectric effect with resultant decreased scatter. The kVp must be high enough, however, to adequately penetrate the patient or else contrast will be severely degraded.

Other factors contributing to overall image contrast include image intensifier quality, inherent film contrast, type of processing, fog, and scatter. Film choice is somewhat determined by individual preference, but in general one should avoid films that have a high level of inherent contrast. Although these films may make "pretty" pictures, some information is invariably lost

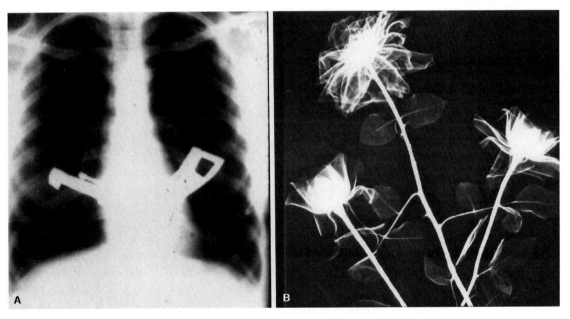

Figure 1-11. Effect of peak kilovoltage (kVp) on image contrast. **(A)** Pistol spirited into the radiology department in the patient's brassiere. The difference in radiographic density between the gun and the patient is easy to understand: they are composed of vastly different materials. **(B)** The small differences in radiographic density among the parts of the roses, all similar in composition, are enhanced by a low-kVp technique.

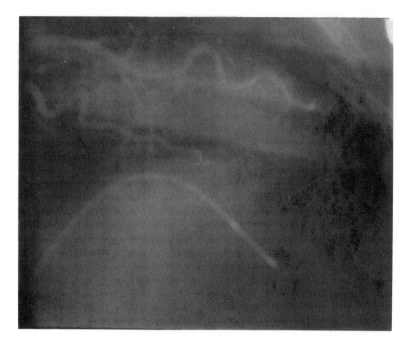

Figure 1-12. Effect of fog on density and contrast. Image density has been increased to beyond acceptable limits by inadvertent exposure of the film to light in the darkroom. As a result, image contrast is also extremely poor.

at the edges of vessels with high contrast techniques. Fog is caused by photographic development of silver crystals on the film that were not exposed to light or exposed to extraneous light. It adds density to the film without providing information and thus decreases contrast (Fig. 1-12). Scatter, described in the previous section, has the same effect as fog on film density and contrast. Scatter can be decreased by using low kVp, decreasing field size, or using a grid.

Resolution

Contrast resolution is the ability to differentiate two objects that have little inherent difference in x-ray absorption characteristics. Angiographic techniques in general have relatively poor contrast resolution. (Computed tomography, on the other hand, has very good contrast resolution.) Spatial resolution is the ability to record separate images of objects placed closely together and is closely related to sharpness, which is the ability to define the edges of those objects. In order to appreciate the factors affecting image sharpness and resolution, some of the causes of unsharpness—quantum mottle, absorption unsharpness,

geometric unsharpness, and motion unsharpness—must be considered.

Quantum mottle is the statistical fluctuation in the number of x-ray photons striking the image intensifier and is the major cause of noise on the x-ray image. The number of x-ray photons in a beam (flux) does not remain constant, even with constant tube current and kVp. Quantum mottle is greater with a low number of photons and decreases as the flux increases. Quantum mottle is readily recognized on radiographs as a salt-and-pepper appearance or graininess (Fig. 1-13). The major cause of quantum mottle is an x-ray dose that is too low. This inadequacy may be built into the system in an ill-advised attempt to decrease the radiation dose to a minimal level, or it may result from the use of high kVp techniques. Because of the way in which cine generators control exposure, quantum mottle increases with large patients and with many of the angled views, particularly the caudal left anterior oblique view (see Chap. 3). There is a level of flux below which adequate imaging is not possible no matter how sophisticated the equipment, and the smaller the object imaged, the higher this flux level will be.

Absorption unsharpness is caused by the shape

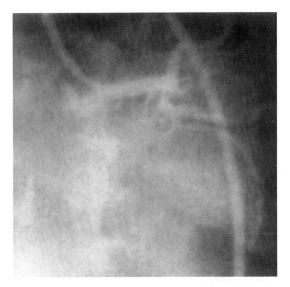

Figure 1-13. Quantum mottle. Caudal posteroanterior view of the left coronary artery in an obese patient shows a grainy image with poor contrast as a result of low photon flux and high kVp.

of the object being imaged. From a radiographic standpoint, all objects should be trapezoidal in shape so that extremely sharp edges could be seen. Unfortunately, very few coronary arteries have that shape, so attenuation of x-rays is usually not uniform across a vessel. As a result, the edges of coronary arteries are always blurred

to some degree, regardless of the quality of the radiograph (Fig. 1-14). Even quantitative angiographic analysis systems must deal with this phenomenon and somewhat arbitrarily choose what to consider as the vessel edge (see Chap. 5).

Geometric unsharpness (penumbra) results from the geometry of the x-ray beam. X-rays do not travel from the target in a parallel fashion but diverge. Furthermore, they do not arise from an infinitely small point on the target but rather from a group of points collectively known as the focal spot. The focal spot has a finite size that ranges from 0.3 to 1.2 mm in most x-ray tubes used for cineangiography. As a result, even if an object has a sharply defined edge, the image of the object will have an edge that consists of an area rather than a line. This area, known as the penumbra, increases with increased size of the focal spot, with decreased distance between the focal spot and the image intensifier, and with increased distance between the object and the intensifier (Fig. 1-15).

For a practical demonstration of this phenomenon, hold a pencil point in front of the light source of a movie or slide projector. Start with the pencil against the screen and notice how the image of the pencil becomes progressively blurred as the distance between the pencil and the screen is increased. Now punch a tiny hole in a piece of opaque paper and place it in

Figure 1-14. Absorption unsharpness. The object being imaged on the left conforms to the shape of the x-ray beam, resulting in an abrupt change in radiographic density at its edge. The circular object on the right has a gradually changing thickness, resulting in a slow increase in radiographic density at the edges of the image.

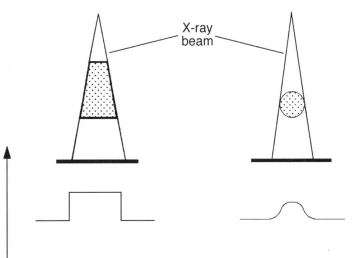

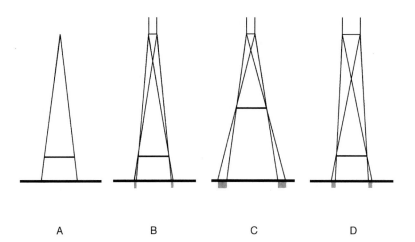

A   B   C   D

Figure 1-15. Penumbra (geometric unsharpness). **(A)** The x-ray beam comes from a (hypothetical) point source, resulting in a very sharp image edge. **(B)** Because the focal spot is not a point source, an image is generated by each point on its surface. This results in multiple image edges, represented here by the gray area on either side of the image. **(C)** Moving the patient closer to the x-ray tube results in a larger object-to-image distance, greater magnification, and greater penumbra. **(D)** Increasing the size of the focal spot also increases penumbra.

front of the light source. The pencil can be moved much farther away from the screen before significant blurring occurs. An analogous situation arises during coronary angiography. Moving the pencil away from the screen corresponds to moving the image intensifier away from the chest wall (increasing object-to-intensifier distance), and placing the pinhole in front of the light source is the same as selecting a smaller focal spot. An unwanted side effect of using the pinhole in the pencil example was a marked decrease in the intensity of the light. Likewise, a small focal spot tolerates a much lower tube current than a large one, necessitating an increase in kVp, pulse width, or both.

Motion unsharpness is caused by movement of the object being imaged. Coronary arteries move at a fairly rapid clip, sometimes as much as several centimeters per second. If the patient is breathing, a second source of motion is added. Short of causing asystole, we cannot do much about coronary motion, but respiratory motion can and should be minimized on every cine run by having the patient stop breathing during the run, preferably at end-inspiration.

One should distinguish between intraframe and interframe motion. The former is motion that occurs during an individual exposure and causes degradation of the image. The latter is motion of the object between frames; it results in a jerky appearance of the angiogram. Some angiographers film at 60 frames per second to decrease interframe motion. Although this results in a smoother-appearing angiogram, the price paid in terms of exposure (at least double) and x-ray factors (high kVp or long exposure time) is often high. Intraframe motion can be minimized by using short pulse widths. A typical cine generator is programmed with pulse widths between 2.5 and 10 msec. Although this may sound like a very short time, 10 msec is one-hundredth of a second, a relatively slow exposure time for imaging a moving object.

WAYS TO IMPROVE IMAGE QUALITY

With the preceding background we can now discuss how a knowledge of the factors affecting cine quality can be used to improve angiographic quality. The goal is to maintain kVp in the range of 70 to 80 kV while keeping exposure time shorter than 8 msec and using a small focal spot. How well this goal is achieved depends both on how the equipment has been set up and how cine factors under the angiographer's direct control are chosen.

There are several parameters that are programmed into the generator when it is installed and can be changed if necessary. The first of these is *exposure per frame*, which is usually expressed as microRoentgens (µR) per frame. Newer systems with highly efficient image intensifiers require less radiation than older systems, but, as mentioned previously, there is a limit below which quality pictures cannot be obtained because of lack of x-ray photons. There is no clear distinction between too few and enough photons, but as a general rule with newer systems, exposure should be maintained at about 15 to 20 µR per frame for 6- or 7-inch (15- or 18-cm) modes, with lower and higher doses for 9- and 5-inch (23- and 13-cm) modes, respectively. If the exposure is set too high, generator workload and tube heating are increased, image quality deteriorates, and radiation exposure is increased for both operator and patient.

Another consideration is maximum programmed *cine run time*. If the maximum run time is programmed to be 15 or 20 seconds, the generator assumes that each run will last that long and chooses the x-ray factors accordingly. Because a long run time results in great tube heating, the kVp is usually set for a higher level to minimize heating. Decreasing the maximum run time to a more reasonable 8 or 10 seconds allows the tube to generate considerably more heat and come nearer to its full kilowatt rating. Because actual run times rarely exceed 6 to 8 seconds, this is a very efficient way to improve x-ray factors at no cost.

A major factor in determining kVp is choice of *focal spot*. Because small focal spots cause less penumbra (see Fig. 1-15), exclusive use of the small focal spot to increase spatial resolution would seem to be desirable. The tube has a lower kilowatt rating when the small focal spot is used, however, which allows less heat loading. This must be compensated by increasing kVp to some degree, creating a dilemma: the angiographer must decide whether to use the large focal spot or use a higher kVp. There are no hard-and-fast rules, but considering the decreased

radiographic contrast associated with beam energies greater than 90 to 100 kVp, switching to the large focal spot may be the better choice if the kVp exceeds that level and exposure time is 8 msec or more on the small focal spot.

Cine *frame rate* also plays an important part in image quality, because the total heat generated by a cine run depends on the number of exposures. A frame rate of 60 frames per second generates about twice the heat as does a rate of 30 frames per second. Therefore, a significant price is paid for the image smoothness that is obtained with higher frame rates—namely, higher kVp and higher x-ray exposure of both patient and operator. For most cardiac applications, 30 frames per second is more than adequate. The faster frame rate should be reserved for pediatric cases and for small adults with heart rates greater than 120 beats per minute.

Pulse width or exposure time has a direct effect on x-ray factors by affecting the mAs. Higher mAs allows for lower kVp but generates proportionately more heat. Furthermore, longer exposure times result in more motion unsharpness. For coronary angiography, pulse widths in the range of 4 to 6.4 msec provide a good compromise between motion unsharpness and tube heating. Pulse width should preferably be limited to 8 msec or less, and in no circumstance should it exceed 10 msec. Similarly, pulse widths shorter than 2.5 msec do not significantly improve motion unsharpness and may result in unacceptably high kVp.

Because the inherent radiographic contrast between blood in the coronary arteries and the myocardium is extremely low, the addition of iodinated *radiographic contrast material* to the blood is required for imaging. Despite this fundamental truth, one frequently encounters underfilled coronary arteries. We facetiously refer to this problem as "thenar palsy syndrome," in recognition of the role of underinjection of contrast material by the person operating the syringe. Other causes are possible, however, such as poor flow distal to a high grade obstruction and high flow states such as seen with hypertension, aortic stenosis, and aortic regurgitation, especially if small-diameter catheters are used. Underfilling of the coronaries can cause several unwanted effects, such as inadequate exposure, underestimation of vessel size, and underestimation of stenoses. Contrast material is usually well tolerated; if there is concern about hemodynamic instability, a nonionic agent can be used to minimize untoward hemodynamic effects. I do not advocate giving huge and unnecessary doses of contrast material, but the patient is not done any favor by sparing the contrast and spoiling the pictures.

A second consideration in choice of contrast material is *iodine concentration*. The standard for many years with ionic contrast media has been 370 mg of iodine per milliliter. Several of the newer agents have lower concentrations; for example, iogloxate is used at only 320 mg/mL. Although this may not make a noticeable difference when kVp is optimal, it clearly affects image quality adversely at higher beam energies (Fig. 1-16). It makes sense to use the agent with the highest concentration of iodine available, and there are low osmolar agents with iodine concentrations of 350 mg/mL and higher. Mixing of blood with contrast material in the syringe should be minimized because it not only decreases iodine concentration but may contribute

to clot formation if nonionic contrast material is used.

The geometry of the x-ray beam has a significant effect on image quality as well. As discussed in the section on geometric unsharpness, an increase in the distance between the heart and the image intensifier causes an increase in penumbra (see Fig. 1-15). This is one reason why the intensifier should be kept as close to the patient's chest wall as possible. Another adverse effect of leaving the intensifier away from the chest wall is the increase in radiation required because of the *inverse square law*. The inverse square law states that exposure varies inversely with the square of the distance between the x-ray source and the image. If the source-to-image distance doubles, the exposure must be quadrupled to maintain constant film density. This has obvious implications in terms of heat loading. A third undesirable effect is the increase in radiographic magnification that occurs with increased distance between the object and the image (Fig. 1-17). When less of the object fits in the intensifier field, more panning is necessary, and motion unsharpness may be increased.

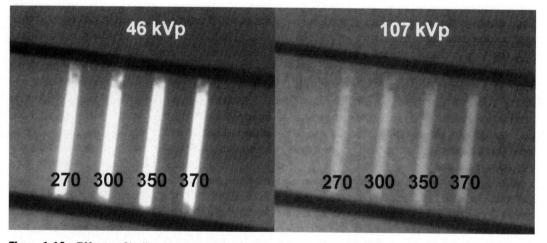

Figure 1-16. Effects of iodine concentration and peak kilovoltage (kVp) on resolution and contrast. Precision-drilled holes in a Plexiglas phantom have been filled with contrast material diluted to various concentrations of iodine (in mg/mL), as indicated on each. The radiograph on the left was taken at 46 kVp and shows sharp images of each hole, with no discernible difference in density among them. The radiograph on the right was taken at 107 kVp and shows a noticeable deterioration in image quality across the board, but with more image degradation at lower iodine concentrations.

A final consideration is that of *field uniformity*. There is a circular area of the image intensifier that serves as a sensing area for the automatic brightness control of the generator. This area usually occupies the central 40% or so of the intensifier. Overall average density in this region is monitored by the generator, and exposure is adjusted accordingly. A great disparity of densities within the sensing area (e.g., the presence of both lung and spine) may result in one area being overexposed and the other underexposed (Fig. 1-18). A similar problem can occur at the edge of the heart, where the cardiac mass is less. Vessels running along the edge may be overexposed as the brightness control tries to penetrate the central cardiac mass. Some of these problems can be avoided by judicious positioning, collimation, and panning; however, the main defense is the *contour collimator*. This is a semiradiolucent collimator made of Plexiglas or other material which can be positioned over the edge of the heart to help even out the difference in density between the heart and the lung. These come in at least two varieties, a single straight shield and dual shields curved to approximate the shape of the heart. Either type can be rotated

and moved in or out as necessary. It is important not to leave the contour collimators in place if they are not needed, because unwanted density will be added to the film, degrading the image. This can be a problem with some shields because they cannot be seen very well unless they are being moved. The value of the contour collimator cannot be overstated, and it is the author's opinion that every catheterization laboratory should have this option.

SUMMARY

Cineangiographic quality is determined by a complex mix of factors, including size and shape of the patient, condition of the x-ray equipment, radiographic technique, and angiographic technique. This chapter provides some of the background information necessary to understand the radiographic side of the equation. As angiographic technique is discussed in the following chapters, it will become apparent how much poor radiographic technique can adversely affect cine quality. By the end of these discussions, all

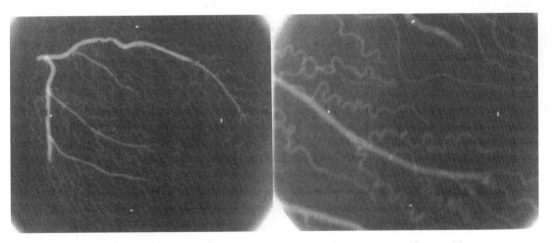

Figure 1-17. Coronary artery phantom showing the effect of image intensifier position (object-to-image distance) on magnification and spatial resolution. In the radiograph on the left, the phantom was placed against the image intensifier, resulting in a similar image with excellent spatial resolution. In the radiograph on the right, the phantom was placed near the x-ray tube. Although larger, the image is considerably less sharp.

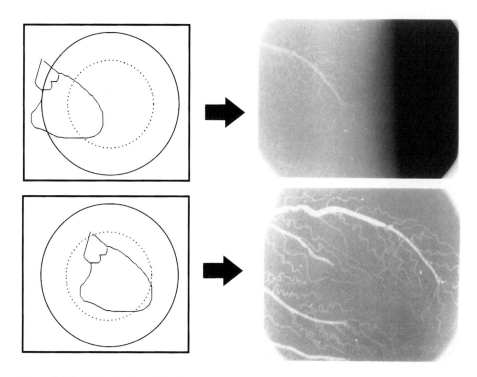

Figure 1-18. Effect of positioning on exposure. The solid circles show the image intensifier size. The dashed circles show the area monitored by the automatic brightness control (ABC). The upper set of images show the results of poor positioning of the phantom; both heart and lung are included in the ABC sensing area. This has resulted in underexposure on the left side and overexposure on the right side. The lower set of images show proper positioning, which results in proper exposure of the heart.

of the relevant factors should come together to explain why some cineangiograms "sparkle" and others are lackluster.

BIBLIOGRAPHY

Culverwell RH: Radiographic imaging techniques for cardiology. In: Elliott LP, ed. Cardiac imaging in infants, children, and adults. Philadelphia, JB Lippincott, 1991:90.

Curry TS, Dowdey JE, Murry RC: Christensen's physics of diagnostic radiology. 4th ed. Philadelphia, Lea & Febiger, 1990.

Coronary Cinematography, by Curtis E. Green.
Lippincott–Raven Publishers, © 1995.

CHAPTER *TWO*

Normal Coronary Anatomy and Variations

The heart is supplied by the right and left coronary arteries, which usually originate from the right and left sinuses of Valsalva, respectively. The posterior sinus rarely gives origin to a coronary artery and is referred to as the noncoronary sinus. The sinuses are not exactly accurately named; however, the right sinus is actually almost anterior in location, and the left is more left and posterior.

The amount of myocardium supplied by each coronary artery is variable, but the right coronary artery (RCA) almost always supplies the right ventricle (RV), and the left coronary artery (LCA) supplies the anterior portion of the ventricular septum and anterior wall of the left ventricle (LV). The supply to the remainder of the LV can be from either coronary artery, depending on the coronary dominance (see Coronary Dominance). Blood supply to the sinoatrial node is from the RCA in a little over half of patients and from the LCA in the remainder. The atrioventricular node is supplied by the RCA in approximately 90% of hearts and by the left circumflex artery (LCx) in the remainder.

RIGHT CORONARY ARTERY

After its origin from the right sinus of Valsalva, the RCA (Fig. 2-1) emerges from under the right atrial appendage to travel in the anterior (right) atrioventricular groove to the crux of the heart (i.e., the junction of the four cardiac chambers). In about half of hearts, the first branch is the *conus artery*, which courses anteriorly to supply the pulmonary outflow tract. In the other half, the conus artery has a separate origin from the aorta. When it arises from the RCA, the *sinoatrial node artery*

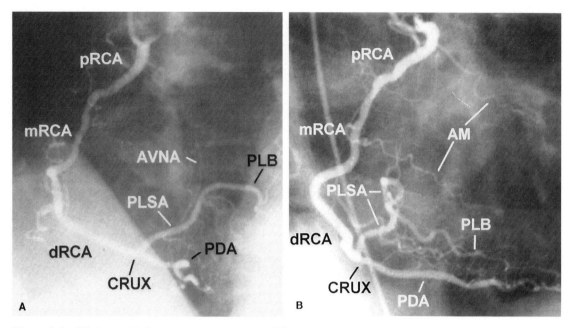

Figure 2-1. (A) Cranial left anterior oblique and **(B)** right anterior oblique views of the right coronary artery. (AM, acute marginal branches; AVNA, atrioventricular node artery; CRUX, crux of the heart; dRCA, distal right coronary artery; mRCA, mid right coronary artery; PDA, posterior descending artery; PLB, posterolateral branch; PLSA, posterolateral segment artery; pRCA, proximal right coronary artery.)

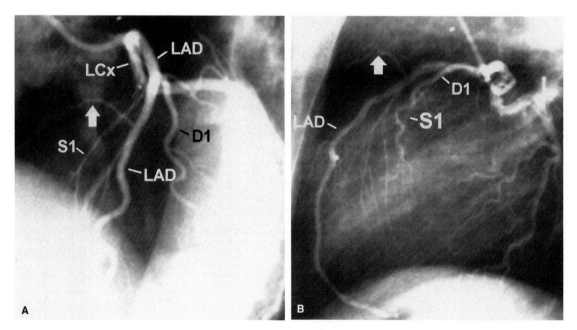

Figure 2-2. (A) Cranial left anterior oblique and **(B)** right anterior oblique views of the left coronary artery showing a right ventricular branch*(arrow)* from the left anterior descending artery (LAD). (D1, first diagonal; LCx, left circumflex artery; S1, first septal perforator.)

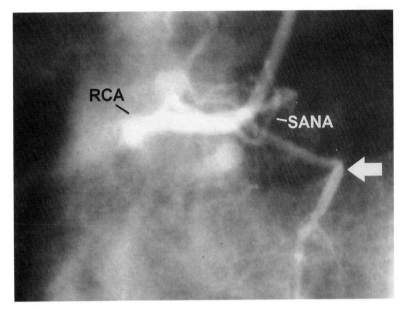

Figure 2-3. Left anterior oblique view of the right coronary artery (RCA) showing a right superior septal perforator *(arrow)*. The septal branch will have an anterior course on the right anterior oblique and lateral views. (SANA, sinoatrial node artery.)

(SANA) is usually the next branch; it courses posteriorly around the superior vena cava in a counterclockwise direction. Frequently, a branch to the atria originates from the SANA. As the RCA goes around the perimeter of the right heart in the atrioventricular groove, it gives off branches that supply the RV myocardium, which are called *right ventricular marginals*, or *acute marginals*. Some observers reserve the term acute marginal for the vessel running along the anterior wall of the RV where it turns into the inferior surface; others use the terms interchangeably. These vessels can be readily identified by their anterior course on the lateral and right anterior oblique views. Chapter 3 contains descriptions of the various coronary angiographic views. Branches from the left anterior descending (LAD) artery can also supply the anterior RV wall (Fig. 2-2). Occasionally, a septal branch comes from the proximal portion

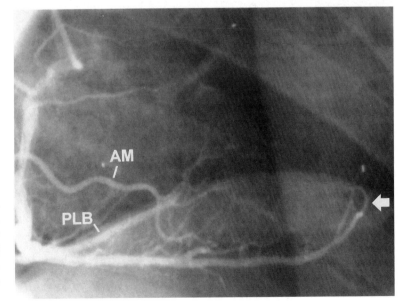

Figure 2-4. Right anterior oblique view of the right coronary artery. The posterior descending artery *(arrow)* reaches the cardiac apex. (AM, acute marginal; PLB, posterolateral branch.)

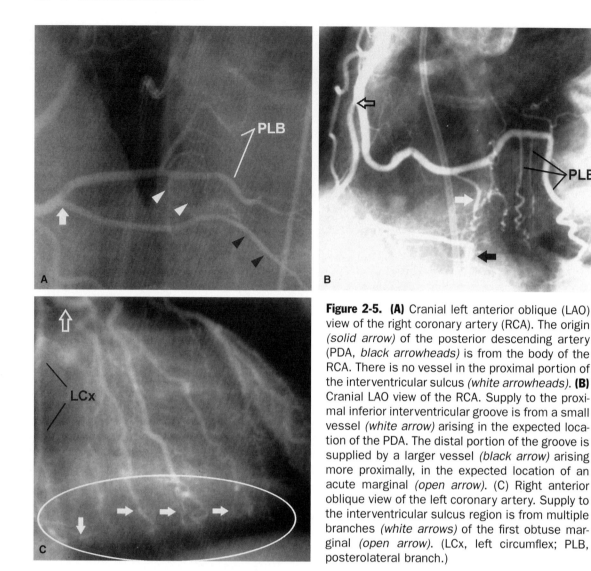

Figure 2-5. (A) Cranial left anterior oblique (LAO) view of the right coronary artery (RCA). The origin *(solid arrow)* of the posterior descending artery (PDA, *black arrowheads)* is from the body of the RCA. There is no vessel in the proximal portion of the interventricular sulcus *(white arrowheads)*. **(B)** Cranial LAO view of the RCA. Supply to the proximal inferior interventricular groove is from a small vessel *(white arrow)* arising in the expected location of the PDA. The distal portion of the groove is supplied by a larger vessel *(black arrow)* arising more proximally, in the expected location of an acute marginal *(open arrow)*. (C) Right anterior oblique view of the left coronary artery. Supply to the interventricular sulcus region is from multiple branches *(white arrows)* of the first obtuse marginal *(open arrow)*. (LCx, left circumflex; PLB, posterolateral branch.)

of the RCA; it is referred to as a *right superior septal perforator* (Fig. 2-3).[1]

The first branch of the RCA to supply the LV is the *posterior descending artery (PDA)*, which courses in the inferior interventricular sulcus to supply the posterior part of the ventricular septum and the diaphragmatic segment of the LV. If it is long enough, it can also supply the apex of the LV (Fig. 2-4). The PDA originates somewhat variably from the distal portion of the RCA, usually just proximal to the crux. It can be difficult to identify with certainty if the septal branches are not apparent and several vessels

course along the diaphragmatic surface of the heart. Variations in PDA anatomy are the rule rather than the exception. Origin from the RCA more proximally in the anterior atrioventricular groove is referred to as early marginal origin of the PDA and is present in a large number of patients, either alone or in combination with a smaller vessel supplying the more proximal portion of the inferior interventricular sulcus (Fig. 2-5A). In this terminology, the word early refers to the fact that the PDA arises early, not to the location of the origin of the acute marginal artery from which it arises. Other variations are also common, including dual PDA with two branches in parallel. Occasionally, the PDA is a diminutive vessel and the LAD wraps around the apex almost to the crux. In other hearts, there is no well-formed PDA, but a group of vessels arising from either the RCA or an obtuse marginal branch of the LCx wrap around the bottom of the heart to supply that region (Fig. 2-5*C*).

Usually arising just distal to the origin of the PDA is the *atrioventricular node artery (AVNA)*, which can be recognized by its vertical course parallel to the body of the RCA. The RCA continues in the posterior atrioventricular groove around the back of the heart as the *posterolateral segment artery (PLSA)* and gives off a variable number of branches, called *posterolateral branches (PLBs)*, which supply the pos-

terolateral wall of the LV. These can be recognized by their course parallel to the PDA.

LEFT CORONARY ARTERY

The LCA normally originates from the left sinus of Valsalva as the *left main (LM) coronary artery*, which soon bifurcates into the *left anterior descending (LAD)* and *left circumflex (LCx)* arteries (Fig. 2-6). In some hearts, the LM is absent, and the LAD and LCx arise from either a common ostium or separate ostia (see Absent Left Main Coronary Artery). The LM runs behind the pulmonary trunk, usually coursing slightly posteriorly at first and then more anteriorly before it bifurcates.

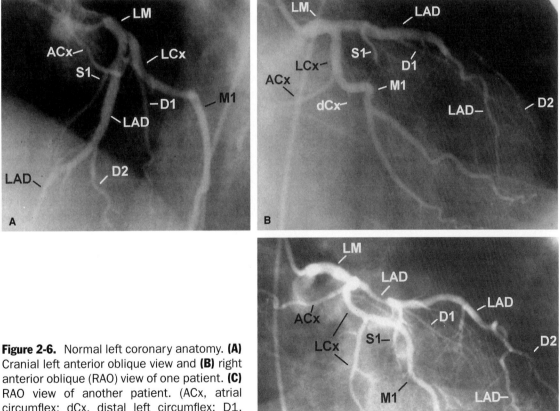

Figure 2-6. Normal left coronary anatomy. **(A)** Cranial left anterior oblique view and **(B)** right anterior oblique (RAO) view of one patient. **(C)** RAO view of another patient. (ACx, atrial circumflex; dCx, distal left circumflex; D1, first diagonal; D2, second diagonal; LAD, left anterior descending; LCx, left circumflex; LM, left main; M1, first obtuse marginal; S1, first septal perforator.)

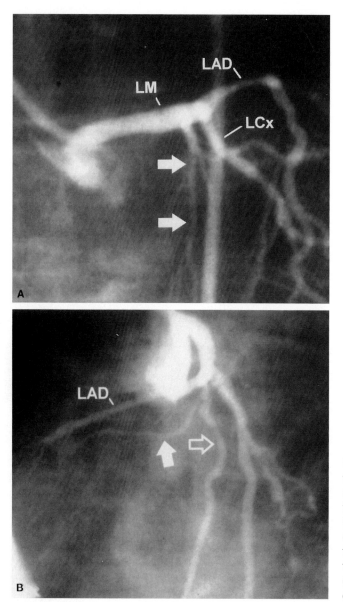

Figure 2-7. (A) Posteroanterior view of the left coronary artery (LCA) showing anomalous origin of the first septal perforator *(solid arrows)* from the left main (LM). **(B)** Cranial left anterior oblique view of the LCA showing anomalous origin of the first septal perforator *(solid arrow)* from the first diagonal *(open arrow)*. (LAD, left anterior descending; LCx, left circumflex).

The LAD runs in the anterior interventricular sulcus directly above the ventricular septum. Its major branches are the *septal arteries*, which run down into the ventricular septum, and *diagonal arteries*, which course over the anterolateral wall of the LV. The LAD usually extends to the apex of the LV, but it can extend around the apex onto the inferior wall of the heart or stop short of the apex. In the latter case, the PDA, a diagonal, or an obtuse marginal supplies the apex. For descriptive purposes, the LAD can be divided into three segments. The proximal segment extends from the origin to the first major septal branch; the remainder of the LAD is divided equally between the mid and distal segments. The diagonals and septals are numbered sequentially (e.g., D1, D2, S1, S2). Septal branches frequently arise from other vessels as well as from the LAD, most commonly from a diagonal, but often from an obtuse marginal or even from the LM (Fig. 2-7).

The LCx runs in the posterior atrioventricular groove toward the PLSA. About 45% of the time, the SANA arises from the proximal LCx, and there is usually a branch to the left atrium that is termed the *atrial circumflex* or *atrial recurrent artery*. The major branches of the LCx are called *left ventricular marginal arteries* or *obtuse marginal arteries* and supply the lateral wall of the LV. They are usually numbered sequentially. The LCx can be divided into segments based on the origins of the marginal arteries, with the proximal segment extending to the origin of the first, the mid segment between the first and second, and the distal segment after the origin of the second marginal. The length of the LCx and the size and number of its marginal branches tend to be inversely proportional to the length of the PLSA and the number of PLBs. They also have a proportional relation to the size and distribution of the first diagonal, because both diagonals and obtuse marginals supply the lateral wall of the LV, and vessels are named by where they come from, not by where they go. It is common to have one very large, obtuse marginal that branches to supply most of the lateral wall (Fig. 2-8). In this case, the distal portion of the LCx is usually either absent or diminutive. The most common variation in LCA anatomy is the presence of a trifurcation of the LM into the LAD, the LCx, and an artery between, called a *ramus intermedius artery* (Fig. 2-9). The ramus can be distributed as either a diagonal or an obtuse marginal depending on whether it goes in front of or behind the left atrial appendage. It is useful to assign it to one of those distributions so as to give the cardiac surgeon some idea of where on the heart to look for it. Keep in mind that the surgeon will be unable to see the origins of many vessels.

CORONARY DOMINANCE

In most patients, the inferior and posterolateral walls of the left ventricle are supplied by the RCA. In a substantial number of patients, however, the LCA makes a significant contribution to the blood supply to these regions. For this reason, it is useful to think in terms of coronary dominance. Although there are several ways to define dominance, the most useful and straightforward is to evaluate the supply to the inferior and inferolateral walls of the LV, because these are the regions with the most variable supply. If the PDA and PLBs arise from the RCA, the system is said to be *right dominant* (see Fig. 2-1); if they arise from the LCA, it is *left dominant* (Fig. 2-10). If the PDA comes from the RCA and the PLBs from the LCA, the system is *codominant* (Fig. 2-11). The reported incidences of left dominant and codominant circulation vary widely depending on how the terms are defined, but one can expect to see right dominance in more than two thirds of patients. In left dominant and codominant systems, the LCx continues in the posterior atrioventricular groove as the *left atrioventricular groove artery (LAVGA)* and gives origin to *left posterolateral branches (LPLBs)*, which are num-

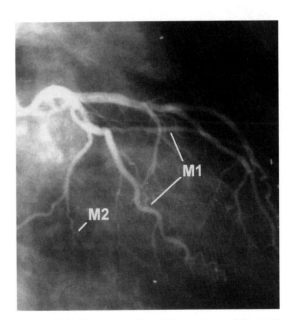

Figure 2-8. Right anterior oblique view of the left coronary artery. Virtually the entire lateral wall of the left ventricle is supplied by branches of the first obtuse marginal (M1). The second obtuse marginal (M2) is tiny.

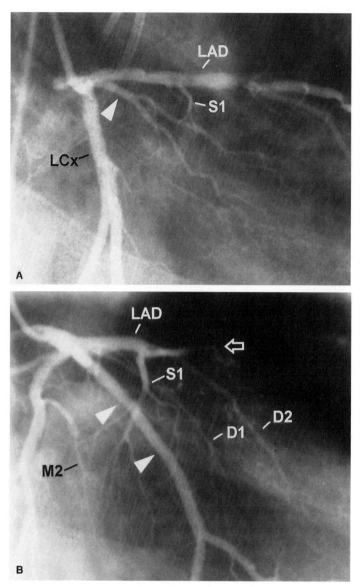

Figure 2-9. Right anterior oblique views of the left coronary artery in two patients. **(A)** The ramus intermedius distributed as a diagonal *(arrowhead)*. **(B)** The ramus intermedius distributed as an obtuse marginal *(arrowheads)*. The left anterior descending (LAD) is occluded *(arrow)* after the origin of the second diagonal (D2). (D1, first diagonal; LCx, left circumflex; M2, second obtuse marginal; S1, first septal perforator.)

bered sequentially from the left. With left dominance, the *left posterior descending artery (LPDA)* is the final branch of the LAVGA, and the AVNA arises just proximal to it (Fig. 2-12). It may be difficult to distinguish left dominant from codominant circulations unless both coronary arteries are visualized. In the case of distal occlusion, the way the coronary vessels curve usually indicates the direction from which they came originally (Fig. 2-12). Sometimes, most of the PLBs come from the LAVGA but one or two small ones originate from the RCA (Fig. 2-13).

Although this makes the circulation technically right dominant, one can think of it as functionally codominant.

For the neophyte angiographer, it can be helpful to think of the coronary arteries as being arranged in a circle and a half-circle or loop (Fig. 2-14). The two atrioventricular grooves form a circle separating the atria from the ventricles; two interventricular sulci form a loop extending from the bottom of the circle to the top. The RCA and LCx run in the circle, and the LAD and the PDA run in the loop.

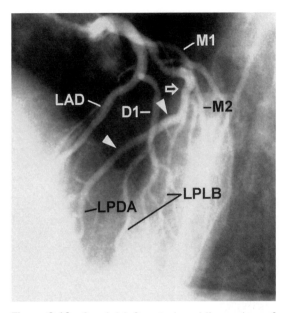

Figure 2-10. Cranial left anterior oblique view of the left coronary artery in a left dominant circulation. The left posterior descending artery (LPDA) and the posterolateral branches (LPLB) arise from the left atrioventricular groove artery *(arrowheads)*, a continuation of the left circumflex *(arrow)*. (D1, first diagonal; LAD, left anterior descending; M1, first obtuse marginal; M2, second obtuse marginal.)

CORONARY ARTERY FISTULAE

Fistulous connections can occur between either coronary artery and the right ventricle, left ventricle (Fig. 2-15*A, B)*, or pulmonary trunk (Fig. 2-15*C)*. Although the literature may imply that these are rare, small fistulae are actually quite common. They are usually of no clinical significance, but if they are large, can cause a significant left-to-right shunt or coronary steal.[2] The fistulae may be fairly discrete, or they may consist of multiple small connections. The involved coronary artery is usually enlarged if the shunt is significant in size. There is some thought that coronary-to-pulmonary fistulae should be ligated to decrease the possibility of rupture or infection, but the necessity of this procedure is not clear-cut.

ANOMALIES OF CORONARY ARTERY ORIGIN

The following discussion is concerned with coronary anomalies that are either common or have major prognostic significance. It is important to be able to recognize these for several reasons. First, although many common anomalies have no physiologic or prognostic significance, they can cause technical problems during the study or lead to misinterpretation of the films. Second, some anomalies are associated with significant morbidity or mortality. This is not intended to be a comprehensive treatise on this subject, and the reader is referred to the excellent reviews by Roberts[3] and by Yamanaka and Hobbs[4] for additional information.

Anomalies of coronary artery origin occur in 0.1% to 0.3% of adults who undergo coronary arteriography. The largest series is that of Yamanaka and Hobbs[4] from the Cleveland Clinic; they found anomalous coronary origins in 1.15% of more than 120,000 patients who underwent diagnostic coronary angiography. In comparison, the group at Texas Heart Institute found an incidence of 0.78% in more than 10,000 patients,[5] and the Coronary Artery Surgery Study group reported an incidence of 0.3% in more than 24,000 patients.[6]

Absent Left Main Coronary Artery

Absent LM (Fig. 2-16) is a relatively common anomaly characterized by either separate ostia or a common ostium for the LAD and LCx. It has no physiologic significance but can cause problems for the angiographer because it is difficult to fill both coronary arteries simultaneously. Also, if this anomaly is not recognized, the films can be misinterpreted as showing occlusion of one of these vessels. If this anomaly is suspected, the best view for confirmation is usually the caudal left anterior oblique view with the catheter at the ostium. A common mistake among both experienced and neophyte angiographers is to try to opacify both the LAD and LCx at the same time. This almost always results in adequate opacification of neither vessel. The best

(text continues on p. 30)

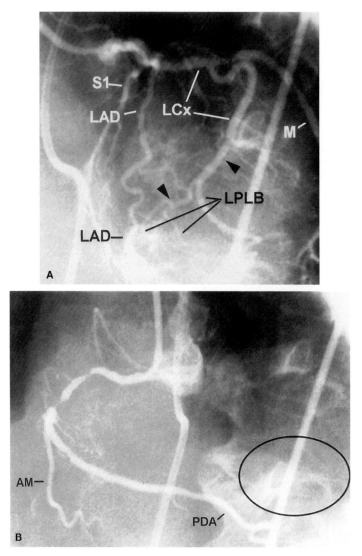

Figure 2-11. Cranial left anterior oblique views of **(A)** the left coronary artery and **(B)** the right coronary artery (RCA) in a codominant circulation. The posterolateral region of the left ventricle is supplied by left posterolateral branches (LPLB) coming from the left atrioventricular groove artery *(arrowheads)*, the continuation of the left circumflex (LCx). The posterior descending artery (PDA) comes from the RCA. No supply to the posterolateral area *(black circle)* comes from the RCA. (AM, acute marginal; LAD, left anterior descending; M, obtuse marginal; S1, first septal perforator.)

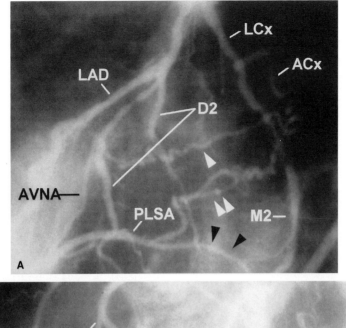

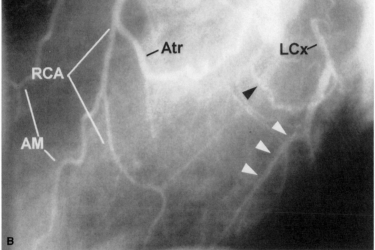

Figure 2-12. (A) Cranial left anterior oblique (LAO) view of the left coronary artery in a right dominant circulation demonstrates collateral filling of an occluded RCA through collaterals from the left circumflex (LCx) to the atrioventricular node artery (AVNA; *single white arrowhead*) and the posterolateral segment artery (PLSA; *double white arrowhead*). Notice how the posterolateral branch *(black arrowheads)* curves back toward the right side of the heart. **(B)** Cranial LAO view of the RCA in a left dominant circulation. Collaterals *(black arrowhead)* from an atrial branch (Atr) of the RCA fill the left posterior descending *(white arrowheads)* which curves back toward the left side of the heart. (ACx, atrial circumflex; AM, acute marginal; D2, second diagonal; LAD, left anterior descending; M2, second obtuse marginal.)

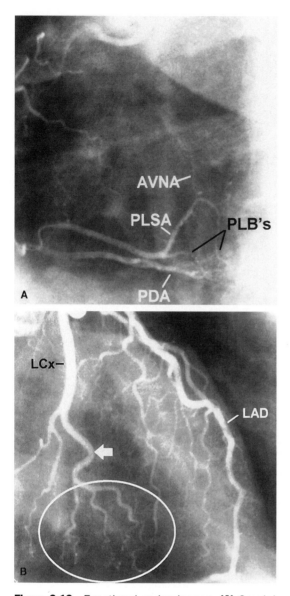

approach is to take selective LAD and LCx angiograms. From an imaging standpoint, this is actually an ideal situation because of far less overlap of vessels than when both are filled at the same time. There are two tricks that can be used to selectively engage the LAD and LCx if it cannot be done with a left Judkins coronary catheter. One is to use a Judkins catheter with a smaller curve. For example, if a No. 4 catheter engages the LAD, a No. 3.5 may engage the

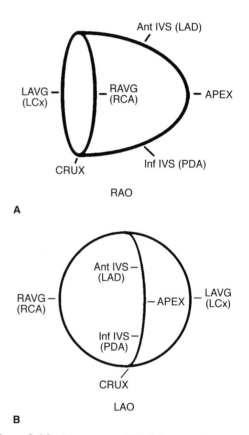

Figure 2-13. Functional codominance. **(A)** Cranial left anterior oblique view of the right coronary artery. **(B)** Right anterior oblique view of the left coronary artery. Although there are some tiny right posterolateral branches (PLBs), the main supply to the posterolateral region of the ventricle *(circle)* comes from branches of an obtuse marginal *(arrow).* (AVNA, atrioventricular node artery; LAD, left anterior descending; LCx, left circumflex; PDA, posterior descending artery; PLSA, postero-lateral segment artery.)

Figure 2-14. Diagrams of **(A)** right anterior oblique (RAO) and **(B)** left anterior oblique (LAO) views of the right (RAVG) and left (LAVG) atrioventricular grooves and the anterior (Ant IVS) and inferior (Inf IVS) interventricular sulci, showing their relations to the major coronary arteries. (APEX, apex of the heart; CRUX, crux of the heart; LAD, left anterior descending; LCx, left circumflex; PDA, posterior descending artery; RCA, right coronary artery.)

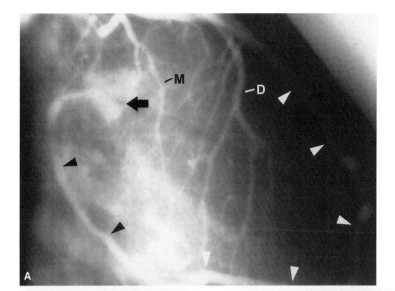

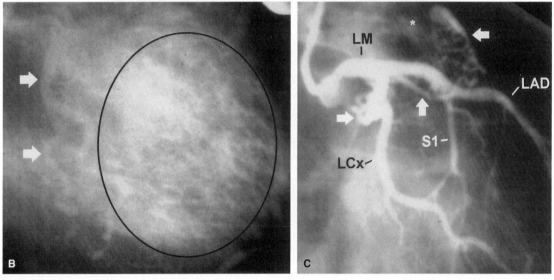

Figure 2-15. Right anterior oblique views of the left coronary artery showing coronary artery fistulae in three different patients. **(A)** There is a very large fistula *(white and black arrowheads)* arising from the left anterior descending (LAD) that enters the left ventricle near the atrioventricular groove *(arrow)*. **(B)** An intense blush is seen over the entire left ventricular cavity *(circled area)* from multiple small fistulae between the LAD and its branches and the ventricle. Contrast material in the left circumflex (LCx; *arrows*) indicates that this view has been made relatively soon after the injection of the contrast agent. **(C)** Fistula *(arrows)* between LCx and the main pulmonary artery *(asterisk)*. (D, diagonal; LAD, left anterior descending; LM, left main; M, obtuse marginal; S1, first septal perforator.)

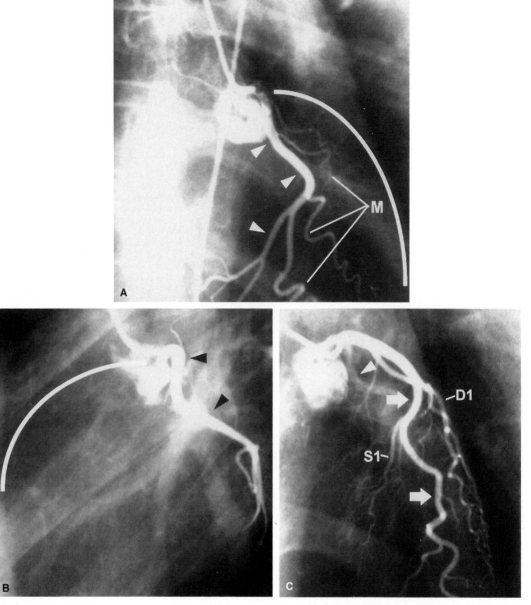

Figure 2-16. (A) Right anterior oblique (RAO) and **(B)** left anterior oblique views of a subselective injection *(arrowheads)* of the left circumflex (LCx). There is no vessel in the expected course *(white line)* of the left anterior descending (LAD). **(C)** RAO view of a subselective injection of the LAD *(arrows)* in the same patient. Flash-filling of the LCx *(arrowhead)* can barely be seen. (D1, first diagonal; M, obtuse marginals; S1, first septal perforator.)

LCx. Alternatively, one can use either a left Amplatz catheter or a multipurpose catheter.

Origin of Coronary Artery From Ascending Aorta

Origin of a coronary artery from the ascending aorta (Fig. 2-17) is uncommon and is usually of no physiologic consequence but can prove to be very difficult to cannulate. The surgeon must be made aware of this anomaly because the coronary could be compromised during cross-clamping of the aorta.

Origin of Left Circumflex Artery From Right Sinus or Right Coronary Artery

Origin of the LCx from the right sinus or the RCA (Fig. 2-18) is the most common major

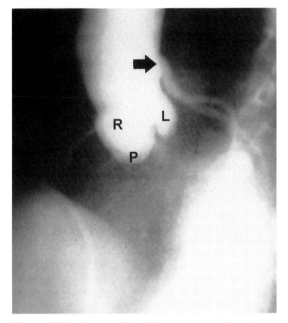

Figure 2-17. Origin of the left coronary artery from the ascending aorta *(arrow)* above the left sinus of Valsalva (L). (P, posterior sinus of Valsalva; R, right sinus of Valsalva.)

anomaly of coronary origin. In most cases, the LCx arises from the RCA itself or from the sinus adjacent to the RCA. Less frequently, it arises from the sinus remotely from the RCA. The course is always posterior to the aorta.[3] This anomaly is fairly easy to miss at angiography because the right Judkins coronary catheter tends to engage the RCA fairly deeply. An anomalous LCx should be suspected if no vessel is present in the left atrioventricular groove. This situation requires a diligent search in the right sinus and sometimes aortography. Origin of the LCx from the RCA is not thought to be associated with symptoms or sudden death. If it arises from the right sinus independently of the RCA, however, a slit-like orifice may be present and could cause ischemia. There is also some evidence that the anomalous LCx is subject to an increased incidence of atherosclerosis. In otherwise matched patients, the Coronary Artery Surgery Study group found a 41% incidence of significant narrowing in anomalous LCx arteries, compared with a 29% incidence in those with normal origins.[6] This difference was not associated with any difference in mortality at 7 years of follow-up, however. It has been hypothesized that the narrowing may be a result of excess tortuosity or of increased turbulence caused by the unusual origin. The major problem caused by this anomaly is misinterpretation of the films as showing an occluded LCx.

Origin of Right Coronary Artery From Left Sinus

Origin of the RCA from the left sinus (Fig. 2-19) is less than half as common as origin of the LCx from the right sinus. The RCA arises from the left sinus, usually above and slightly anterior to the ostium of the LCA, and courses between the aorta and the pulmonary trunk. The clinical significance is unclear. Roberts found no cases of symptoms caused by this anomaly in 26 necropsied patients but found a combined incidence of symptoms or sudden death in 12 of 34 patients reported in other studies.[7] If the anomaly is symptomatic, sudden death is usually not the

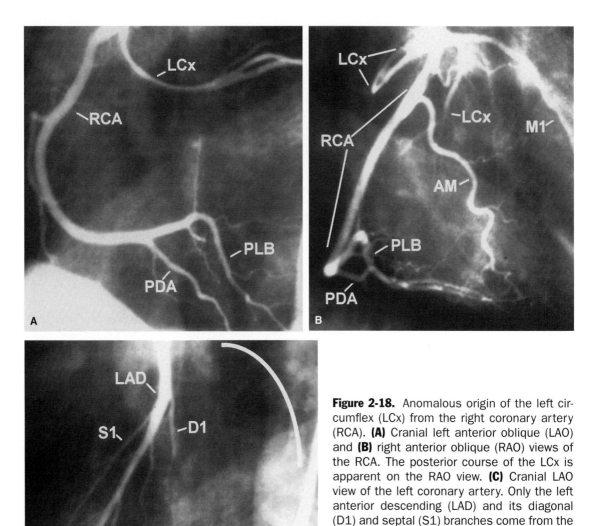

Figure 2-18. Anomalous origin of the left circumflex (LCx) from the right coronary artery (RCA). **(A)** Cranial left anterior oblique (LAO) and **(B)** right anterior oblique (RAO) views of the RCA. The posterior course of the LCx is apparent on the RAO view. **(C)** Cranial LAO view of the left coronary artery. Only the left anterior descending (LAD) and its diagonal (D1) and septal (S1) branches come from the left sinus; there is no vessel in the expected course of the LCx (*curved white line*). (AM, acute marginal; M1, first obtuse marginal; PDA, posterior descending artery; PLB, posterolateral branch; PLSA, posterolateral segment artery.)

initial presentation. Possible mechanisms for ischemia include compression between the aorta and pulmonary artery, stretching around the aorta, and obstruction of the orifice by the unusual angle of origin.[7-11] It may be very difficult to engage the RCA if it arises from the left sinus. Left coronary bypass, multipurpose, and Amplatz catheters can all be used with variable success. As with the anomalous LCx, it is important to have a high index of suspicion if the RCA cannot be engaged and there is neither a stump nor collateral filling from the LCA.

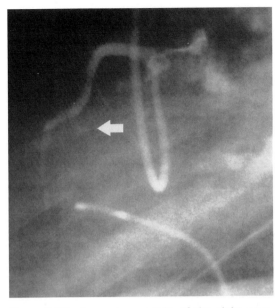

Figure 2-19. Anomalous origin of the right coronary artery (RCA) from the left sinus of Valsalva. Left anterior oblique view shows the origin of the RCA to be above and medial to its usual location *(arrow)*.

Origin of Left Coronary Artery From Right Sinus

Origin of the LCA from the right sinus is about half as common as origin of the RCA from the left sinus, but it is potentially more serious (Fig. 2-20). One study reported a 27% incidence of sudden death in patients with this anomaly.[12] Five different types have been described, depending on the course of the LM and its branches to the left side.[4] The most dangerous course is passage of the LM between the aorta and the pulmonary artery. This can be recognized on the right anterior oblique view as a cranial-anterior course. The LAD and LCx appear to have normal lengths. This anomaly has been associated with angina, sudden death, syncope, myocardial infarction, and ventricular tachycardia, most frequently in young patients during or immediately after exertion. Passage of the LM into the ventricular septum (i.e., the septal course) is more common and is usually not associated with symptoms unless there is

coexisting coronary artery disease. It can be recognized on the right anterior oblique view as a caudal-anterior loop that gives a "hammocked" appearance. The LM can also pass anterior to the pulmonary artery, taking a course similar to that of a conus branch. This condition is also usually benign. Rarely, the LCA courses posterior to the aorta and forms a caudal-posterior loop on the angiogram. Combined forms also exist in which, for example, the LCx passes posterior to the aorta, the septal between the aorta and the pulmonary trunk, and the LAD anterior to the pulmonary trunk.

Single Coronary Artery

Single coronary artery (Fig. 2-21) is probably more correctly referred to as single coronary ostium. It is very rare, especially in the absence of other congenital heart disease. It occurs when the LM and the RCA share a common ostium from the aorta, from either the right or left sinus of Valsalva. The classification suggested by Lipton and colleagues[13] is the least confusing of the nomenclature schemes. In their system, the coronary is first classified according to the sinus from which it arises, either right (R) or left (L). Second, it is placed into a group depending on the basic morphology. If the single coronary follows the course of either a normal right or left coronary artery, it is put into Group 1; if one coronary appears to arise from the proximal portion of the other, it is put into Group 2. Group 3 contains those arrangements that demonstrate combinations of the other two types. For example, if the LCx continues into the anterior atrioventricular groove to supply the entire RCA distribution, it is classified as L1. On the other hand, origin of the LM from the proximal RCA is classified as R2. A third level in this nomenclature describes the course of the transverse branch of the coronary artery, with "a" denoting passage anterior to the pulmonary trunk, "b" denoting passage between the aorta and the pulmonary trunk, and "p" denoting passage posterior to the aorta. This has obvious similarities to the classification used for origin of the LCA from the right sinus. The bottom line

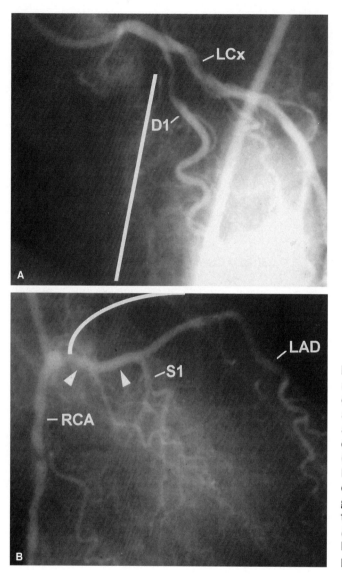

Figure 2-20. Anomalous origin of the left anterior descending (LAD) from the right coronary artery (RCA). **(A)** Cranial left anterior oblique view of the left coronary artery shows no vessel in the expected course of the LAD *(straight white line)*. **(B)** Right anterior oblique view of the RCA. The inferiorly "hammocked" course of the proximal LAD *(arrowheads)* suggests a septal course. Passage between the great vessels would be as shown *(curved white line)*. (D1, first diagonal; LCx, left circumflex; S1, first septal perforator.)

here is the same as for the other anomalies in which a coronary artery arises from the wrong sinus: passage between the great vessels is associated with significant morbidity and mortality.

Origin of Coronary Artery From Pulmonary Artery

Origin of a coronary artery from the pulmonary artery is very rare in adults. The LCA is the most frequently involved artery, but the majority of patients present in infancy with heart failure or ischemia. If there is sufficient shunting of blood from the RCA into the LCA, the patient may survive into adulthood but is still at risk for sudden death.[3] Most of these patients have symptoms of ischemia first, usually with exercise. Origin of the LAD or the RCA from the pulmonary artery is much less common. Patients with pulmonary origin of the RCA are often asymptomatic[14] but can present with coronary

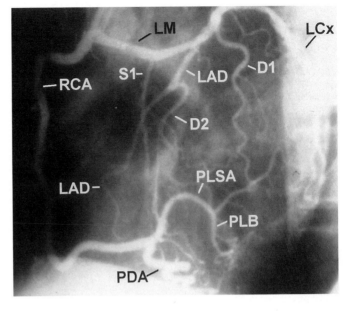

Figure 2-21. Left anterior oblique view of the right coronary artery (RCA) showing anomalous origin of the left coronary from the RCA with the septal course of the left main (LM). (D1, first diagonal; D2, second diagonal; LAD, left anterior descending; LCx, left circumflex; PDA, posterior descending artery; PLB, posterolateral branch; PLSA, posterolateral segment artery; S1, first septal perforator.)

steal.[15] Origin of the LAD from the pulmonary artery is usually associated with angina in adults.[16] If it is present, this anomaly can be identified by injection of the RCA: prompt filling of the LAD and then the pulmonary artery is observed. It is pointless to try to inject the orifice of the LAD from the pulmonary artery; not only is it extremely difficult to find, but the LAD will probably not opacify because blood is flowing in the wrong direction.

REFERENCES

1. Bream PR, Souza AS, Elliott LP, et al. Right superior septal perforator artery: its angiographic description and clinical significance. Am J Roentgenol 1979;133:67.
2. St John Sutton MG, Miller GA, Kerr IH, Traill TA. Coronary steal via large coronary artery to bronchial artery anastomosis successfully treated by operation. Br Heart J 1980; 44:460.
3. Roberts WC. Major anomalies of coronary arterial origin seen in adulthood. Am Heart J 1986; 111:941.
4. Yamanaka O, Hobbs RE. Coronary artery anomalies in 126,595 patients undergoing coronary arteriography. Cathet Cardiovasc Diagn 1990;21:28.
5. Wilkins CE, Betancourt B, Mathur VS, et al. Coronary artery anomalies: a review of more than 10,000 patients from the Clayton Cardiovascular Laboratories. Tex Heart Inst J 1988;15:166.
6. Click RL, Holmes DR, Vlietstra RE, et al. Anomalous coronary arteries: location, degree of atherosclerosis and effect on survival a report from the Coronary Artery Surgery Study. J Am Coll Cardiol 1989; 13:531.
7. Roberts WC, Siegel RJ, Zipes DP. Origin of the right coronary artery from the left sinus of Valsalva and its functional consequences: analysis of 10 necropsy patients. Am J Cardiol 1982;49:863.
8. Benge W, Martins JB, Funk DC. Morbidity associated with anomalous origin of the right coronary artery from the left sinus of Valsalva. Am Heart J 1980;99:96.
9. Brandt B, Martins JB, Marcus ML. Anomalous origin of the right coronary artery

from the left sinus of Valsalva. N Engl J Med 1983;309:596.

10. Isner JM, Shen EM, Martin ET, Fortin RV. Sudden unexpected death as a result of anomalous origin of the right coronary artery from the left sinus of Valsalva. Am J Med 1984;76:155.

11. Bett JHN, O'Brien MF, Murray PJS. Surgery for anomalous origin of the right coronary artery. Br Heart J 1985;53:459.

12. Cheitlin MD, DeCastro CM, McAllister HA. Sudden death as a complication of anomalous left coronary origin from the anterior sinus of Valsalva. Circulation 1974;50:780.

13. Lipton MJ, Barry WH, Obrez I, et al. Isolated single coronary artery: diagnosis, angiographic classification, and clinical significance. Radiology 1979;130:39.

14. Lerberg DB, Ogden JA, Zuberbuhler JR, Bahnson HT. Anomalous origin of the right coronary artery from the pulmonary artery. Ann Thorac Surg 1979;27:87.

15. Mintz GS, Iskandrian AS, Bemis CE, et al. Myocardial ischemia in anomalous origin of the right coronary artery from the pulmonary trunk. Proof of a coronary steal. Am J Cardiol 1983;51:610.

16. Roberts WC, Rabinowitz M. Anomalous origin of the left anterior descending coronary artery from the pulmonary trunk with origin of the right and left circumflex coronary arteries from the aorta. Am J Cardiol 1984;54:1381.

Coronary Cinematography, by Curtis E. Green.
Lippincott–Raven Publishers, © 1995.

CHAPTER *THREE*

Principles of Axial Coronary Angiography

The coronary arteries are small, tortuous, constantly in motion, and highly variable in their distribution and orientation. All of these factors conspire to make them among the most difficult anatomic structures to image. As a result, a great deal of attention must be payed to the technical details of the cineangiograms if diagnostic quality is to be maintained. Chapter 1 described some of the physics of image quality; this chapter addresses issues and problems of anatomy.

The development of axial views is probably the most important advance in coronary angiography since the development of the image intensifier and the replacement of cut film with cine film. There can no longer be any doubt about the absolute necessity of using angled views; numerous studies have demonstrated the gross inadequacy of angiograms that rely only on views limited to rotation in the transverse plane. Axial angiography has not come without a price, however. Equipment workload is increased, study time tends to be slightly longer, and radiation exposure of both patient and operator is higher. Furthermore, angled views require significantly more attention to detail. The rewards easily justify the costs, however, and no knowledgeable angiographer would suggest that diagnostic-quality coronary angiograms can be obtained without triaxial angulation.

TECHNICAL CONSIDERATIONS

As with most other radiographic techniques, an important goal in angiography is to visualize each coronary artery segment from two, preferably orthogonal, directions, perpendicular to the x-ray beam and free of overlapping vessels. It is unlikely

39

that all three of these goals can be achieved in a given patient, but with constant attention to detail, each coronary angiogram can be as close to the theoretical ideal as possible.

Originally, angiographic views were determined by the orientation of the x-ray tubes and were thus limited to anteroposterior and lateral. This equipment configuration had little relation to the orientation of the coronary arteries, and it soon became obvious that rotation in the transverse plane to obtain right anterior oblique (RAO) and left anterior oblique (LAO) views was necessary. This was initially achieved by rotating the patient and keeping the x-ray tubes stationary. Not only was this system uncomfortable for the patient, but it also limited the amount of rotation. The next step was to place the x-ray tube and image intensifier on a rotating gantry and keep the patient stationary.

These refinements resulted in less foreshortening of vessels that run primarily in the transverse plane: the proximal left anterior descending (LAD) artery, the obtuse and acute marginals, the diagonals, the posterior descending artery (PDA), and the posterolateral branches, but did not address the problem of foreshortening of vessels running primarily longitudinally, such as the right coronary artery (RCA), the left circumflex (LCx), and the distal LAD. This problem requires angulation of the beam toward the head or the feet.

In radiographic terms, a view is described based on the path of the x-ray beam. Accordingly, if the beam passes from the feet toward the head, it is said to be caudal-cranial, and if it passes from the head toward the feet, it is termed cranial-caudal. These terms are more readily remembered by abbreviation according to the position of the image intensifier relative to the patient. If the intensifier is near the patient's shoulder, the view is referred to as cranial (Cr; Fig. 3-1A), and if it is near the hip, the view is referred to as caudal (Cd; Fig. 3-1B). The word "angulation" is used in this text to refer to movement in a cranial or caudal direction. The word "rotation" refers to movement in the transverse plane (right or left anterior oblique).

Triaxial angulation can be accomplished in several ways. The cranial views were originally obtained by propping up the patient on a wedge with transverse rotation achieved by either rotating a cradle or rotating the gantry. With some of the earlier C-arm gantries (e.g., Siemens Cardioskop-U, Philips Cardiodiagnost-C), both caudal and cranial angulation could be obtained by swiveling the x-ray table away from or toward the operator. If the gantry were rotated RAO, moving the foot of the table away resulted in cranial angulation, and pulling it toward the operator resulted in caudal angulation. The converse was true for LAO rotation: moving the foot of the table away caused caudal angulation, and pulling it toward the operator produced cranial angulation. The major disadvantage of these systems was that the amount of angulation was dependent on the degree of rotation. For example, with no tube rotation (frontal view), table swiveling results in no angulation. Although angulation was achieved by swiveling the C-arm on its base, the original General Electric LU-C had the same problem. The first popular unit to make use of direct sagittal angulation was the Philips Polydiagnost-C, which uses a parallelogram arrangement. Currently, almost all manufacturers provide a means of obtaining complex angles without moving either the patient or the table.

In coronary angiography, it is often impossible to adequately evaluate the coronary arteries by use of a routine set of views that do not take into account the unique anatomy of each patient. Although certain views are used in almost every patient, constant refinements and adjustments must be made to allow for variations in the origins and courses of the vessels. Although it is faster, a "cookbook" study often results in unanswered questions. Routine views should serve only as the framework on which each study is built.

One of the questions most frequently asked by fellows and by catheterization laboratory personnel concerns the amount of angulation one should use for each view. Although the angles employed usually fall within a fairly narrow range, they must be adjusted on an individual basis. In general, 60 to 90 degrees of LAO and 30 to 45 degrees of RAO rotation are used. Cranial and caudal angulations are usually in the

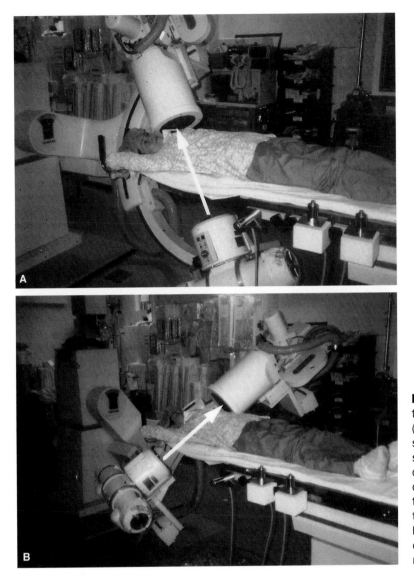

Figure 3-1. **(A)** Cranial positioning, left anterior oblique (LAO) view. The image intensifier is over the subject's shoulder; the x-ray beam comes from near the hip and courses in the direction of the arrow. **(B)** Caudal positioning LAO view. The x-ray beam comes from the shoulder; the image intensifier is near the hip.

range of 20 to 30 degrees but occasionally are greater. The factors that determine the exact amount of angulation necessary include the orientation of the heart, the ability of the patient to breathe, the orientation of the coronary arteries, and the technical capability of the x-ray equipment.

It is important to consider the capability of the x-ray equipment. The potential amount of caudal and cranial angulation advertised in sales brochures (usually 45 degrees) is frequently unobtainable with a patient on the table unless

one is willing to sacrifice the patient's cranium or the x-ray tube (Fig. 3-2). Furthermore, extremely angulated views may require output in excess of what the generator and tube are capable of producing. This is especially true in larger patients, for whom one must frequently temper the desire to use high-magnification mode and shallow, highly angulated views.

The x-ray gantry rotates about a point in space which is called the *isocenter*. If the center of the heart (the object of interest in this case) is at isocenter, no matter which way the gantry is

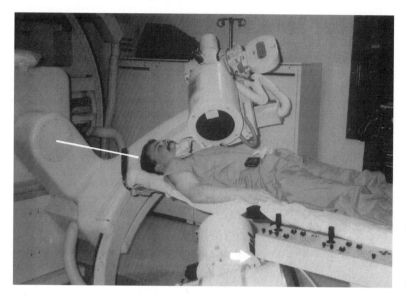

Figure 3-2. Cranial left anterior oblique (LAO) view. At 50 degrees of LAO rotation, the maximum amount of cranial angulation achievable is 33 degrees. At that point, the x-ray tube impinges on the control box *(arrow)*. The patient is at isocenter, as indicated by the line running parallel to the table from the pivot point of the image intensifier to the middle of the body.

rotated, the heart will be in or near the center of the x-ray field (Fig. 3-3*A, B*). Because coronary angiography deals with a fairly small field (usually 5—9 inches [15—23cm] wide), this is a major consideration. The heart can readily be placed at isocenter by centering it in the x-ray field with the gantry vertical, then rotating the gantry to left lateral (90-degree LAO rotation) and, without moving the table from side to side, raising or lowering the table so that the heart is centered in the field. If this is done properly, it should not be necessary to make much lateral adjustment with the table in any view unless the heart is very large or high-magnification mode is used. If the heart is not at isocenter, it is difficult to adequately position it in the image field or pan satisfactorily (Fig. 3-3*C, D*).

Systems that allow both the table and the gantry to move up and down give the angiographer more flexibility but also create the opportunity for more confusion. If the operator has to repeatedly adjust the table and move the gantry up and down to get the heart in the field, the heart is almost certainly out of isocenter. Raising the table and the intensifier, which places the heart above isocenter, sometimes allows a few more degrees of cranial angulation (Fig. 3-4). The price for this adjustment is twofold: higher equipment workload because of greater distance

between the x-ray tube and the image intensifier (i.e., source-to-image distance), and inability to pan all over parts of the heart. If the angiographer then forgets to put the heart back in isocenter, the next view may be a complete disaster. During biplane filming, it is critical to have the heart at isocenter for both planes, or one plane will not include the areas of interest (see Fig. 3-3*C, D*).

VIEWS FOR THE LEFT CORONARY ARTERY

Posteroanterior View

The left main coronary artery usually originates from the left sinus with a posterior orientation, usually about 120 degrees from the sagittal plane, and then curves anteriorly. A schematic based on the data of McAlpine[1] is shown in Figure 3-5. As a result, the straight frontal or posteroanterior (PA) view is generally the most useful for evaluation of the body of the left main coronary artery (Fig. 3-6*A*). The origin and bifurcation of the left main coronary artery are usually best seen in the 30-degree LAO and shallow RAO views, respectively, because they

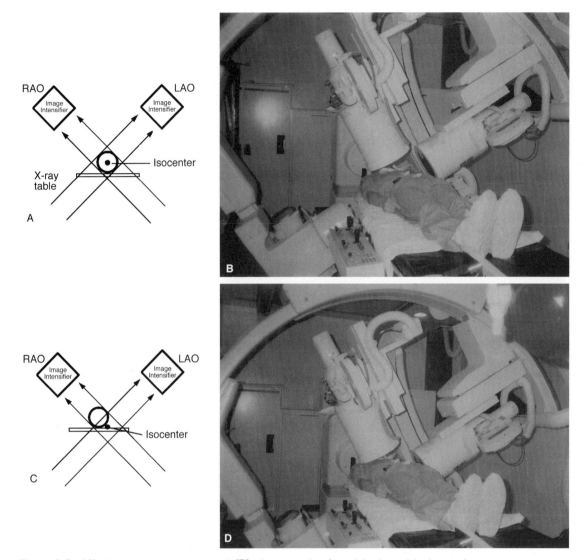

Figure 3-3. (A) Schematic diagram and **(B)** photograph of positioning with the patient isocentered. The heart, represented by the large circle, is within the x-ray field in both right anterior oblique (RAO) and left anterior oblique (LAO) views. **(C)** Schematic diagram and **(D)** photograph of positioning with the patient above isocenter. The table has been pulled toward the operator, which has positioned the heart within the x-ray field in the RAO view; however, it is out of the field in the orthogonal (i.e., LAO) view.

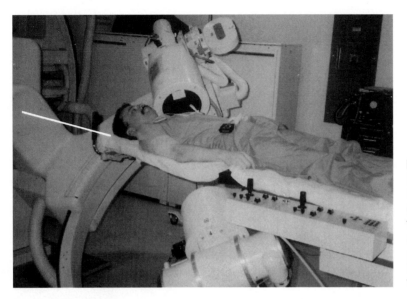

Figure 3-4. Fifty degrees of left anterior oblique positioning. Extra cranial angulation (43 degrees) has been obtained by raising the subject above isocenter. (The line parallel to the table is now below the subject). Compare with Figure 3-2.

are more or less orthogonal to these parts of the artery. The PA view is actually a shallow LAO view with just enough rotation so that the catheter is not superimposed on the left main coronary artery (usually 10—15 degrees). This unfortunately places the vessel directly over the spine, but that is unavoidable because further LAO rotation and slight RAO rotation result in foreshortening (Fig. 3-6B). Either caudal or

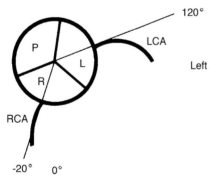

Figure 3-5. Schematic diagram of the orientation of the coronary ostia showing the average orientation of the origins relative to the sagittal plane. The average left coronary ostium is therefore profiled in a 30-degree left anterior oblique (LAO) view and the average right coronary ostium in a 70-degree LAO view.

cranial angulation can be added if there is any suspicion of an eccentric lesion. Caudal angulation also serves to open the bifurcation better,[2] but it can result in image degradation because of higher peak kilovoltage (kVp) and increased quantum mottle (Fig. 3-7A). Most of the advantages of caudal angulation in the PA view can be obtained with the caudal RAO view. The cranial PA view has been used to delineate the proximal and mid portions of the LAD and the origins of the diagonal arteries for angioplasty (Fig. 3-7B). Exposure may be less than ideal, however, because of inclusion of the spine and the diaphragm in the field.

Cranial Left Anterior Oblique View

Originally described by Bunnell as the "half-axial view,"[3] the cranial left anterior oblique (Cr-LAO) view was essentially the first axial view used in coronary angiography. It is an important view for looking at the origin and bifurcation of the left main coronary artery, the proximal portions of the LAD and LCx, and the origins of the diagonals (Fig. 3-8), and it is far superior to the straight LAO view for viewing these areas (Fig. 3-9A, B). In left dominant systems, it is also useful for evaluating the PDA and left posterolateral branches. Traditionally, about 60

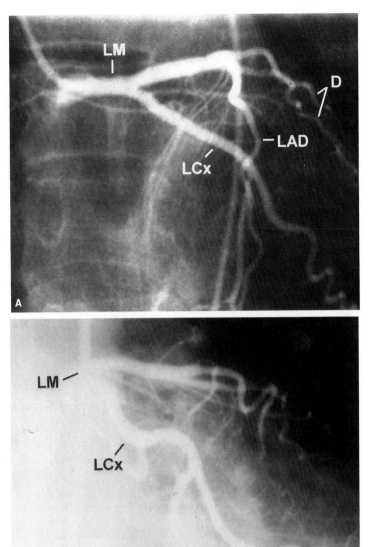

Figure 3-6. (A) Posteroanterior view of the left coronary artery. Even though the left main (LM) is over the spine, the uniform x-ray field results in satisfactory exposure of all areas of interest. **(B)** Shallow (20-degree) right anterior oblique view of the left coronary artery. The LM is grossly foreshortened. Because of the gross differences in the densities of the spine, heart, and lung, the area over the spine is underexposed while that over the border of the heart is overexposed. (D, diagonal arteries; LAD, left anterior descending; LCx, left circumflex.)

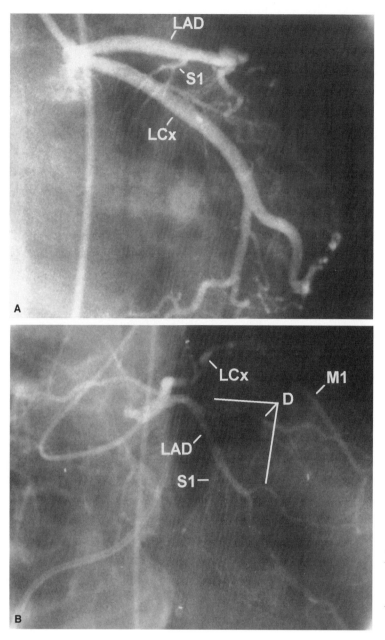

Figure 3-7. (A) Caudal and **(B)** cranial posteroanterior views of the left coronary artery. (D, diagonal arteries; LAD, left anterior descending; LCx, left circumflex; M1, first obtuse marginal; S1, first septal perforator.)

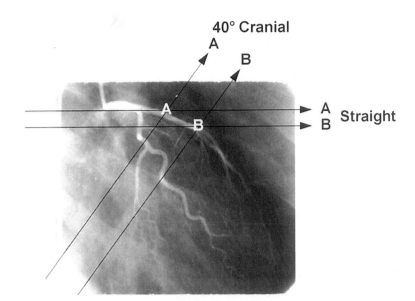

Figure 3-8. Right anterior oblique view of the left coronary artery showing the projected paths of the x-ray beam in cranial and straight left anterior oblique (LAO) views. Imagine the image intensifier to be on the right side of the illustration and the x-ray tube to be on the left side with the beam passing from left to right in the direction of the arrows. The projection seen will be orthogonal to that shown; that is LAO. The distance between points A and B is substantially greater with 40 degrees of cranial angulation than in the straight LAO view.

degrees of LAO rotation and 25 degrees of cranial angulation have been used (Fig. 3-9B, C). This provides good separation of the LCx and LAD and keeps the LCx from overlapping the spine but has two disadvantages: the distal LAD is superimposed on the diaphragm, and the origins of the diagonals may overlap the LAD. This has led some angiographers, particularly interventionalists, to use less LAO rotation (i.e., 30–40 degrees), frequently with more cranial angulation (Fig. 3-9D). Although this solves the problem of diagonal-LAD overlap, the distal LAD overlaps both the spine and diaphragm, and the LCx is over the spine. If the patient is large, these areas may be seriously obscured (Fig. 3-9E). The choice of the "standard" Cr-LAO view or this "exaggerated" Cr-LAO view should be determined on the basis of the area of interest. In general, the standard view is superior for the average diagnostic study, and the exaggerated view is more useful for LAD and diagonal angioplasty work.

Most patients do not require contour collimation for the Cr-LAO view of the left coronary artery (LCA) because the vessels of interest are on the side of the heart away from visible lung. If a shield is necessary (e.g., if the right coronary artery [RCA] fills by collaterals), it should be placed just over the right side of the heart.

Caudal Left Anterior Oblique View

The caudal left anterior oblique (Cd-LAO) view supplements the Cr-LAO view in patients with a horizontal or upgoing left main coronary artery[4] (Fig. 3-10). This is most likely to occur in obese patients, particularly those with limited respiratory excursion. Under these circumstances, the proximal LAD is likely to be foreshortened and the left main bifurcation poorly seen in the Cr-LAO view (Fig. 3-11A). To achieve the most from the Cd-LAO view, two things must happen. First, the LAD must not be superimposed

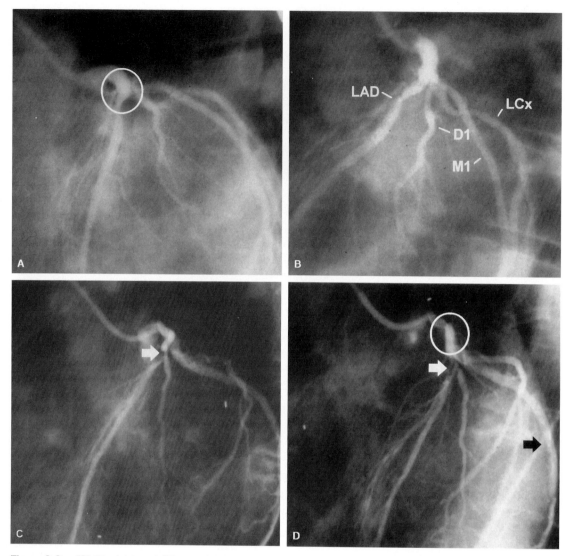

Figure 3-9. **(A)** Straight and **(B)** standard cranial left anterior oblique (LAO) views of the left coronary in a single patient. There is substantial foreshortening of the proximal portion of the left anterior descending (LAD) *(area within white circle)*, and the distal left (LM) is obscured on the straight view. In the cranial view, the first diagonal (D1), left anterior descending (LAD), left circumflex (LCx), and first obtuse marginal (M1) are better defined, and the distal LM is visible. **(C)** Standard and **(D)** shallow cranial LAO views in a second patient. The lesion in the proximal LAD *(white arrow)* is seen much better in the shallower view; however, the proximal LAD and proximal LCx overlap *(circle)*. Although the LCx *(black arrow)* is over the spine, it is adequately exposed in this thin patient.

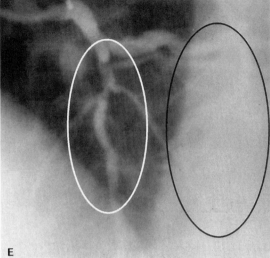

Figure 3-9. (E) Shallow cranial LAO view in a large patient. The only vessels that are seen well are the mid LAD and the diagonal origins *(area within white oval)*; the LCx is over the spine and underexposed *(area within black oval).*

on the left main coronary. This can be accomplished by using enough LAO rotation to bring the lateral wall of the left ventricle just clear of the spine, usually about 60 degrees (Fig. 3-11B). Shallower views with the heart over the spine frequently obscure the bifurcation of the left main (Fig. 3-11C). Second, the upsloping course of the left main must be exaggerated as much as possible. This is achieved by having the patient completely exhale. A deep breath negates the caudal angulation and should never be used.

Unfortunately, the Cd-LAO view comes with a high price tag from a radiographic and radiation perspective. Radiographic factors are less optimal than in almost any other view, resulting in a great deal of scatter and quantum mottle owing to the high kVp necessary to adequately penetrate larger patients. Because of this, the nonmagnified 9-inch (23-cm) mode must occasionally be used to allow adequate film exposure (see Fig. 3-11B). If the generator does not allow filming because of underexposure, another trick is to center the x-ray field over the lung initially

Figure 3-10. Right anterior oblique view of the left coronary in a patient with horizontal left main and left anterior descending arteries. The projected paths of the x-ray beams in straight and cranial left anterior oblique (LAO) views are shown. Ninety-degrees of cranial angulation, a physical impossibility, would be necesary to adequately visualize these vessels in the LAO projection (see Figure 3-8).

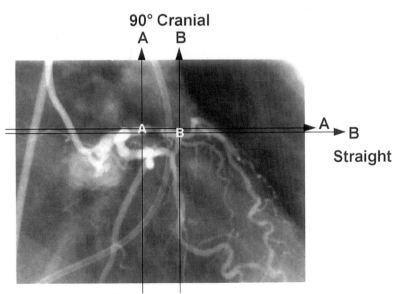

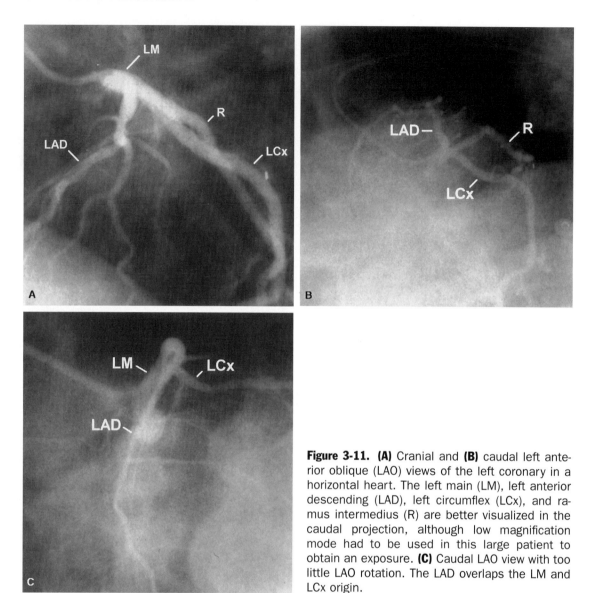

Figure 3-11. (A) Cranial and **(B)** caudal left anterior oblique (LAO) views of the left coronary in a horizontal heart. The left main (LM), left anterior descending (LAD), left circumflex (LCx), and ramus intermedius (R) are better visualized in the caudal projection, although low magnification mode had to be used in this large patient to obtain an exposure. **(C)** Caudal LAO view with too little LAO rotation. The LAD overlaps the LM and LCx origin.

and then pan down onto the heart (Fig. 3-11*D, E*). This results in some degree of underexposure, but at least an exposure is obtainable. Shielding is never necessary in this view and in fact should be studiously avoided, because any extraneous density may further compromise image quality. If the heart is vertical in orientation, the Cd-LAO view is not useful (Fig. 3-12) and should be omitted.

Left Lateral View

Although it is underappreciated and underutilized, the straight lateral view can provide important information. It complements the Cr-LAO view by allowing visualization of the distal LAD free of the diaphragm and the LCx free of the spine (Fig. 3-13*A*). It also usually allows for better visualization of the obtuse marginals,

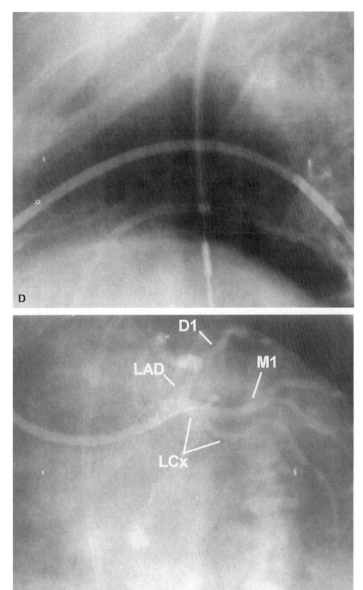

Figure 3-11. (D) and **(E)**. "Fooling" the automatic brightness control by setting up the shot over the lung and panning down onto the heart. Although underexposed, the origins of the main vessels are fairly well seen. (D1, first diagonal; M1, first obtuse marginal.)

which are foreshortened and superimposed on the LCx in the Cr-LAO view. In some cases, the lateral view is useful for distinguishing between the LAD and a large diagonal or marginal that reaches the apex (Fig. 3-13B, C), especially if there is a large septal perforator that could be mistaken for the LAD in the cranial LAO view.

There are three important considerations in setting up and panning in the lateral view. First, the patient's arms must be placed above his or her head to prevent misexposure and extraneous radiodensity. Second, panning in this view requires both dropping the table and moving it to the left (i.e., toward the gantry). Pushing the

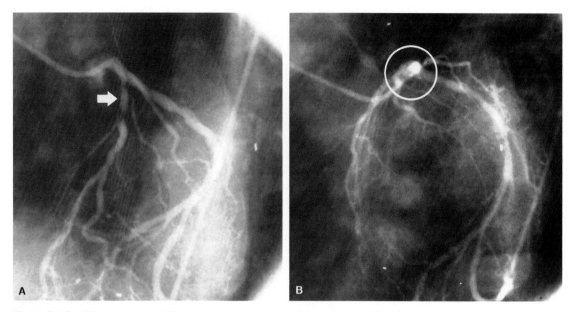

Figure 3-12. **(A)** Cranial and **(B)** caudal left anterior oblique views of the left coronary in a patient with a vertically oriented heart. The proximal left anterior descending *(arrow)* is seen well in the cranial view but is severely foreshortened in the caudal view *(area within circle).*

table away or pulling it toward the operator does not affect the position of the heart in the field but merely changes magnification. The motions should be deliberate and as limited as possible: the sternum does not need to be radiographed. If medium magnification mode is used and the heart is properly positioned, little panning is necessary for most hearts, perhaps just slightly to the left and then a little down (see Fig. 3-13*B*). Third, the contour collimator or shield should be positioned obliquely across the anterior wall of the left ventricle, just over the course of the LAD.

Cranial Lateral View

The cranial lateral view is usually reserved for cases in which the LAD and LCx are superimposed proximally in the Cr-LAO view and the bifurcation of the left main is obscured in the lateral view. In vertically oriented hearts, this may be the only view that profiles the origin of a ramus intermedius artery or an early-arising diagonal. Occasionally, mid LAD or diagonalesions are better seen (Fig. 3-14) with the cranial lateral view.

Straight Left Anterior Oblique View

When a true lateral view is technically unfeasible because of equipment limitations or because the patient's arms cannot be placed above the head, a 60-degree straight LAO view may provide similar information. It usually does not add much new information to the study otherwise, but it may be useful in evaluating the LCx (see Fig. 3-9*A*).

Right Anterior Oblique View

The RAO view is a good view for overall evaluation of the LCA because the x-ray factors are usually good and it is easy to become oriented to the anatomy (Fig. 3-15*A*). On the downside, the proximal LCx is almost always foreshortened, and the LAD and diagonals are frequently superimposed. Thirty to 40 degrees of RAO tube rotation usually works well. Less rotation adds the spine to the field and foreshortens the LAD and obtuse marginals (see Fig. 3-6); more rotation increases the kVp and also foreshortens the same vessels. It is also important to shield the upper edge of the heart adjacent to the

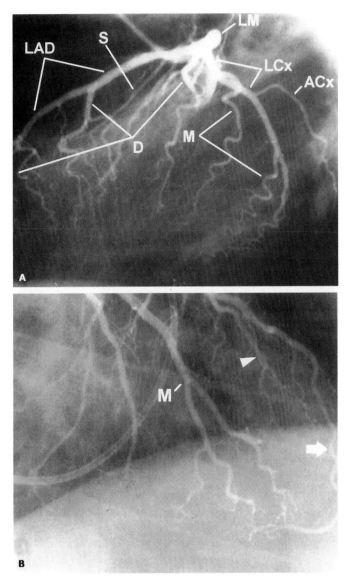

Figure 3-13. (A) Properly positioned lateral view of the left coronary. **(B)** Cranial right anterior oblique view shows what appears to be a large left anterior descending (LAD) reaching the apex *(arrow)*. A smaller vessel *(arrowhead)* appears to be a diagonal. *(continued)*

LAD, because the heart is thinner in this region and vessels along the edge would otherwise be overexposed.

Caudal Right Anterior Oblique View

Adding caudal angulation to the RAO view decreases the foreshortening of the proximal LCx (Fig. 3-16) and allows better visualization of the origin and proximal portion of the LCx[5] (Fig. 3-17) Because of this fact, it can be considered one of the two most important views of the LCA, the other being Cr-LAO view. If a

ramus intermedius artery is present, its origin is also better seen with the Cd-RAO than with the straight RAO view. This improvement in visualization of the proximal LCx and of early obtuse marginal or ramus artery origins does not extend to the distal LCx and more distal obtuse marginals, however. Because they run primarily in the transverse plane, foreshortening of the obtuse marginals is most affected by tube rotation, not angulation. In some patients, the LAD and diagonals are also well seen, but not as consistently as with the Cr-RAO view. The major disadvantage of the Cd-RAO view is degradation of image quality caused by greater exposure

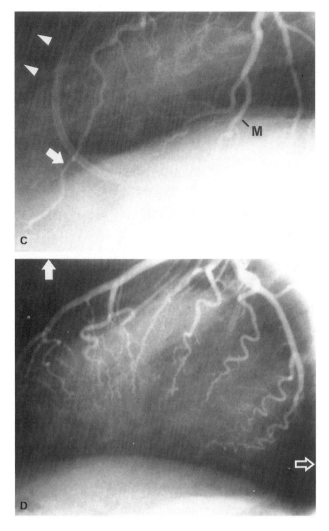

Figure 3-13. *(Continued)* **(C)** Lateral view reveals the larger vessel *(arrow)* to be a diagonal and the smaller vessel *(arrowheads)* to be the LAD. Failure to use a contour collimator has resulted in overexposure of the LAD. **(D)** Panning in the lateral view. Moving the table toward the operator's left results in movement of the left coronary toward the top of the field *(solid arrow)*; posterior movement *(open arrow)* is achieved by dropping the height of the table. (ACx, atrial circumflex; D, diagonal arteries; LCx, left circumflex; LM, left main; M, obtuse marginal; S, septal perforator.)

factors than those required by either the straight or Cr-RAO views. From a practical perspective, this means that during coronary angioplasty, it is usually better to use the straight RAO view for looking at lesions in the body of an obtuse marginal or in the distal parts of the LCx, because there is less quantum mottle and better radiographic contrast (Fig. 3-18).

Cranial Right Anterior Oblique View

Unlike most views, which reveal one area best but can be useful for other vessels as well, the cranial right anterior oblique (Cr-RAO) view looks almost exclusively at the LAD, the diago-

nals, and the origins of the septal perforators[6] (Fig. 3-19A). The LCx is severely foreshortened, and the obtuse marginals are frequently superimposed in this view. The Cr-RAO view was originally described with about 30 degrees of RAO rotation, 25 degrees of cranial angulation, and full inspiration (see Fig. 3-19A); however, there are several variations that may be useful depending on the exact area of interest and the orientation of the coronary arteries. One useful trick is to have the patient suspend respiration instead of taking a deep breath. This effectively increases the amount of cranial angulation and, in some patients, improves separation of the LAD and diagonals, although at the price of superimposition of the distal LAD over the

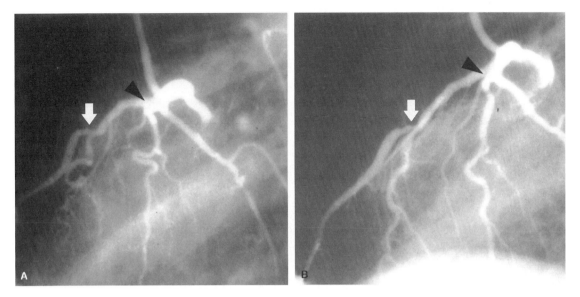

Figure 3-14. (A) Lateral and **(B)** cranial lateral views of the left coronary. Both the stenosis in the mid left anterior descending *(white arrow)* and the origin of the ramus intermedius *(black arrowhead)* are better seen in the cranial view in this patient.

diaphragm (Fig. 3-19*B*). This may not be a problem, however, because the distal LAD is usually well seen in the straight RAO view. Full expiration further exaggerates this effect (Fig. 3-19*C*) but can lead to less-than-satisfactory x-ray technique. Unless the entire LAD and all the diagonals are overlapping the diaphragm, a contour collimator must be used to prevent gross underexposure of the portion of the LAD

that is not over the diaphragm. If the Cr-RAO view is taken with a full inspiration, x-ray factors are usually good, even in large patients.

Occasionally, it is useful to use less RAO tube rotation, perhaps as little as 10 to 15 degrees, with as much cranial angulation as possible and full expiration. Although this method often clearly reveals the diagonal origins and the proximal part of the LAD, new information is not

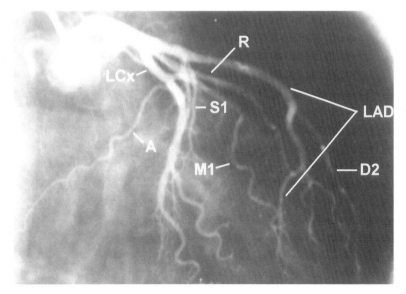

Figure 3-15. Right anterior oblique view of the left coronary. (A, atrial branch; D2, second diagonal; LAD, left anterior descending; LCx, left circumflex; M1, first obtuse marginal S1, first septal perforator; R, ramus intermedius.)

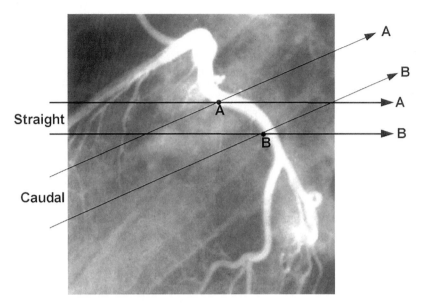

Figure 3-16. Left anterior oblique view of the left coronary showing the projected paths of the x-ray beam in straight and caudal right anterior oblique views. The beam is more perpendicular to the left circumflex in the caudal view, resulting in a greater projected distance between points A and B than in the straight view. Compare with Figure 3-8.

usually gained, and this technique should probably not be used routinely because radiographic factors and image quality tend to be suboptimal (Fig. 3-20).

In evaluating the LCA, it should be remembered that sometimes the RCA fills by means of collateral arteries and must be evaluated at the same time (see Fig. 3-19B). The Cr-RAO is also one of the most important views for the distal RCA branches.

Philosophy of Angiography of the Left Coronary Artery

One goal of coronary angiography is to gain the most amount of information using the least amount of contrast material and radiation. This goal should not be met at the expense of diagnostic accuracy, however. With certain exceptions, most patients deserve a minimum set of views of the LCA. These should include PA, Cr-LAO, lateral, RAO, Cr-RAO, and Cd-RAO views, supplemented with others as necessary

and tailored to the individual's anatomy. Some special views are excellent for looking at specific areas for intervention but are poor choices for the average diagnostic study. These include the exaggerated Cr-LAO, the shallow Cr-RAO and the cranial PA views. Because one can usually tell whether a Cd-LAO view will be necessary by looking at the Cr-LAO and straight RAO views, it does not need to be done routinely. If it is necessary to minimize the number of shots because of left main disease, hemodynamic instability, or critical aortic stenosis, the Cr-LAO and Cd-RAO views should be taken first, because they usually give the most information.

VIEWS FOR THE RIGHT CORONARY ARTERY

The RCA is usually substantially less difficult to evaluate than the LCA because there are fewer branch vessels involved. This translates into fewer views in most patients.

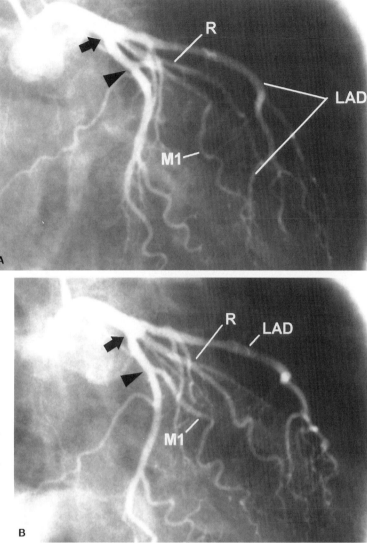

Figure 3-17. (A) Straight and **(B)** caudal right anterior oblique views of the left coronary. The distance between the orgin of the left circumflex *(arrow)* and the origin of the first obtuse marginal *(arrowhead)* is greater in the caudal view, indicating less foreshortening than in the straight view. (LAD, left anterior descending; M1, first obtuse marginal; R, ramus intermedius.)

Lateral View

The lateral view of the RCA is probably the most neglected view of either coronary artery. This is unfortunate, because the anteriorly placed ostium of the RCA[1] (see Fig. 3-5) is usually well visualized in the lateral view, and the body of the RCA is projected clear of the right ventricular (acute) marginal branches without foreshortening (Fig. 3-21). Also, because considerably more tube rotation is used than is usually the case with the Cr-LAO view, a different look at the body of the RCA and the origin of the PDA is obtained than with the cranial view. From a technical standpoint, catheter engagement in the lateral

view is as easy or even easier than in the LAO view, because the ostium is profiled better.

Left Anterior Oblique View

Unless made with the heart clear of the spine, which usually requires 60 or more degrees of LAO rotation, the straight LAO view is inferior to the lateral view in almost all respects: the ostium is not as well profiled, the acute marginals may be superimposed on the body of the RCA, and the PDA is more foreshortened. Furthermore, the amount of rotation may be so similar to that of the Cr-LAO that little addi-

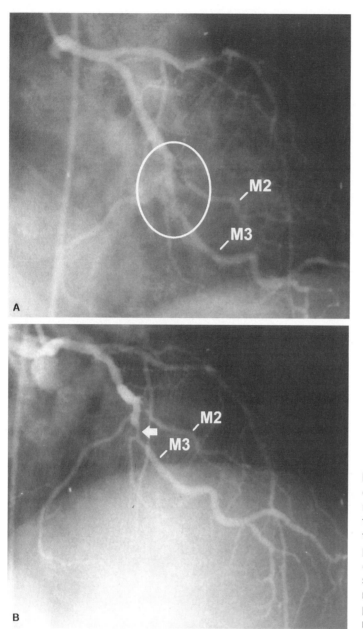

Figure 3-18. **(A)** Caudal right anterior oblique (RAO) view of the left coronary. The distal left circumflex and the origins of the second (M2) and third (M3) obtuse marginals are poorly defined (*area within white circle*.) **(B)** Cranial RAO view demonstrate the stenosis (*arrow*) much more clearly, as a result of lower peak kilovoltage, with less quantum mottle and better contrast.

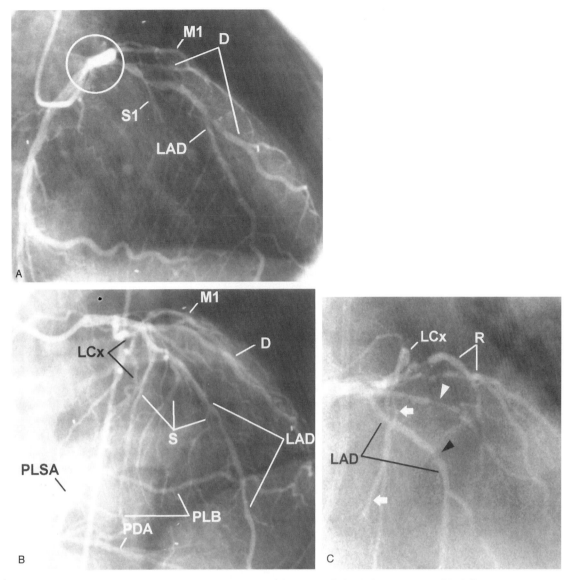

Figure 3-19. (A) Cranial right anterior oblique (RAO) view of the left coronary with full inspiration shows the origins of the first two diagonals (D) and the first septal perforator (S1) free of the left anterior descending (LAD). The first obtuse marginal (M1) is projected above the LAD. **(B)** Cranial RAO view with suspended respiration in a different patient. Separation of the LAD and the diagonal is exaggerated. Collateral filling of an occluded right coronary is present. Less RAO rotation has been used than in **A**. **(C)** Cranial RAO view with full exhalation. The LAD and its branches are well separated; however, superimposition of the vessels on the diaphram has resulted in a noisy image with poor definition of lesions in the mid LAD *(black arrowhead)* and first diagonal *(white arrowhead)*. Notice the anomalous origin of the first septal perforator *(white arrows)* from the first diagonal. (LCx, left circumflex; PDA, posterior descending artery; PLB, posterolateral branch; PLSA, posterolateral segment; R, ramus intermedius; S, septal perforators.)

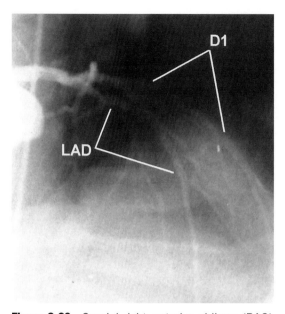

Figure 3-20. Cranial right anterior oblique (RAO) view with 15 degrees of RAO rotation, 35 degrees of cranial angulation, and full exhalation has resulted in gross overexposure of the left anterior descending (LAD) and first diagonal (D1). This view could have been partially salvaged by positioning the image intensifier more over the lung and using a contour collimator.

tional information is gained except that the body of the RCA is not foreshortened (Fig. 3-22). About the only advantage of using the LAO view instead of a lateral view is that the patient's arms do not need to be placed above the head. This seems like a small benefit at a potentially high cost in image quality. Some angiographers tend to use a shallow LAO view for catheter engagement before adding more LAO rotation for the angiogram. The disadvantage in this approach is that if the pressure damps, there will be considerable temptation to inject immediately, even if the view is not what was initially planned. Because even an occluded RCA can provide collaterals to the LCA, there will be a risk of not seeing these collaterals because of superimposition of the LCA on the spine with resultant underexposure.

Cranial Left Anterior Oblique View

The Cr-LAO view is the best view for opening the crux and evaluating the PDA and postero-

lateral branches, which are less foreshortened than in the straight LAO view. It requires adjustment of the amount of tube rotation so that the PDA is projected into the clear space between the spine and the diaphragm (Fig. 3-23A). When too much LAO rotation is used, the PDA is superimposed on the diaphragm (Fig. 3-23B); with too little, it is over the spine (Fig. 3-23C, D). This view should not be used in place of a lateral or straight LAO view because there is substantial foreshortening of the body of the RCA, which can lead to underestimation of lesions in that region. If the angiographer uses the Cr-RAO view as the only other view of the RCA, this problem is compounded.

In setting up and panning the Cr-LAO view, one must be cognizant of the presence of the diaphragm in the x-ray field. It is difficult for the automatic brightness control to properly expose the heart with both lung and diaphragm in the field. This requires some thought as to the initial position. If too much diaphragm is included

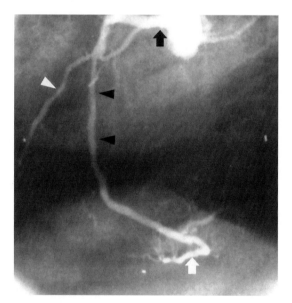

Figure 3-21. Lateral view of the right coronary artery (RCA). The origin of the RCA *(black arrow)* is optimally visualized, and the body of the RCA *(black arrowheads)* and the acute marginal branch *(white arrowhead)* are well separated. Although the posterior descending *(white arrow)* is foreshortened, its origin is seen well.

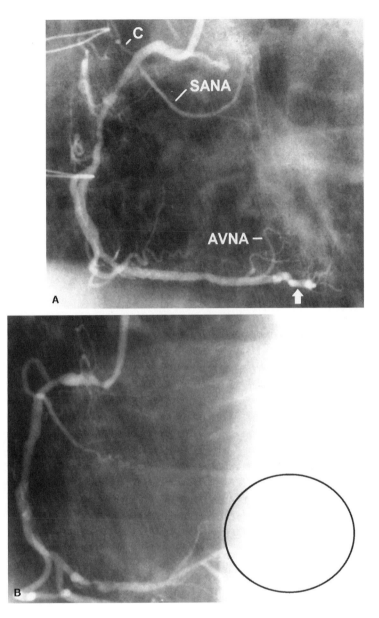

Figure 3-22. (A) Left anterior oblique (LAO) view of the right coronary with 60 degrees of LAO rotation projects the entire vessel clear of the spine. **(B)** Use of 30 to 40 degrees of LAO rotation results in superimposition of the posterolateral wall of the left ventricle *(area within circle)* over the spine. (AVNA, atrioventricular node artery; C, conus artery; SANA, sinoatrial node.)

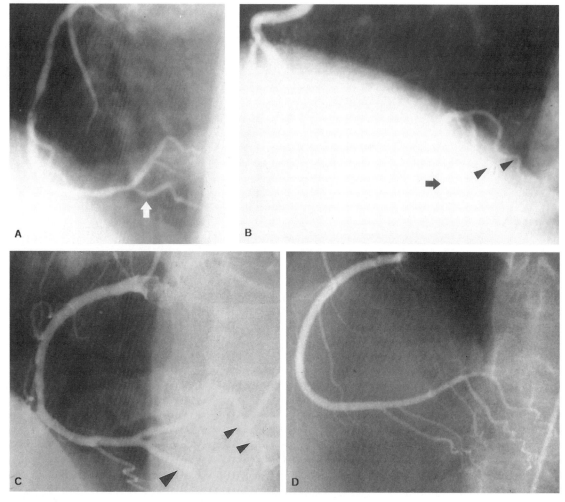

Figure 3-23. **(A)** Properly positioned cranial left anterior oblique (LAO) view of the right coronary artery (RCA) with the posterior descending artery (PDA, *arrow*) projected into the clear space between the spine and the diaphragm. **(B)** More LAO rotation has resulted in superimposition of part of the RCA over the diaphragm. Although the two posterolateral branches *(arrowheads)* are seen, the region of the PDA *(arrow)* is underexposed, and it cannot be seen. **(C)** Slightly less LAO rotation than in **A** has resulted in projection of the PDA *(large arrowhead)* and posterolateral branches *(small arrowheads)* over the spine. **(D)** Shallow LAO view with extreme cranial angulation. Adequate exposure in this case was achieved because of proper positioning, which excluded lung from the field, and small patient size.

initially, the upper portion of the RCA will be overexposed; if too much lung is included, the generator will not have sufficient reserve to penetrate the diaphragm after panning. Placement of the PDA in the clear area between the spine and the diaphragm significantly decreases this problem.

Right Anterior Oblique View

Although some angiographers omit the straight RAO view from routine studies of the RCA, it has two major advantages over the Cr-RAO view: the body of the RCA is not as foreshortened, and the x-ray factors are better because the distal branches are not superimposed on the diaphragm (Fig. 3-24A). The most important disadvantage to this view is that the PDA and the posterolateral branches may be superimposed. It is obvious when this has occurred, because fewer vessels can be seen in the RAO view than were visible in the Cr-LAO. If branches of the LCA fill from right collaterals, the RAO is frequently the best view because of its generally good x-ray factors.

It is important to use a moderate amount of rotation, usually 25 to 30 degrees. This projects the posterolateral segment artery (PLSA) in front of the body of the RCA so that the origins of the posterolateral branches are not superimposed on the PLSA. More rotation also foreshortens the PDA and posterolateral branches (Fig. 3-24B).

One further consideration is that the origin of the RCA is never visualized in the RAO view. This can be a factor if the initial LAO or lateral view shows what is thought to be catheter-induced spasm and nitroglycerin is given to confirm that impression. If the next view is an RAO of any sort, the question will remain unanswered. This may seem obvious, but it is actually a relatively common mistake, even among experienced angiographers.

Cranial Right Anterior Oblique View

The Cr-RAO view is useful if the distal branches of the RCA, the PDA and posterolateral branches, are superimposed in the RAO view.[6]

(text continues on p. 67)

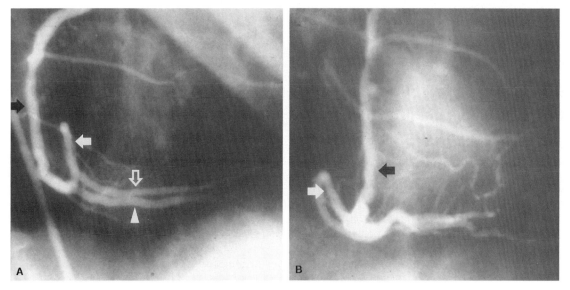

Figure 3-24. (A) Right anterior oblique (RAO) view of the right coronary artery (RCA) with 25 degrees of RAO rotation. The posterolateral segment artery (PLSA, *solid white arrow*) is projected in front of the body of the RCA *(black arrow)*. The posterior descending artery (PDA, *arrowhead*) and the posterolateral branch (PLB, *open arrow*) are barely separated. **(B)** Forty-degree RAO view of the RCA in the same patient. The PLSA *(white arrow)* is now projected behind the body of the RCA *(black arrow)*, causing foreshortening of the PLB. Futhermore, the PDA and PLBs are now completely superimposed.

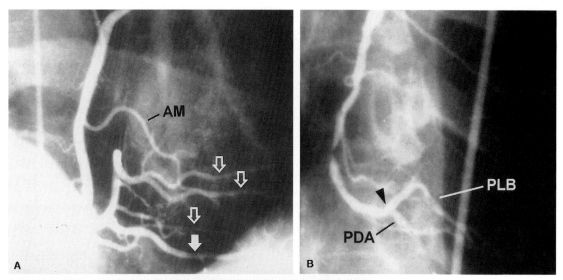

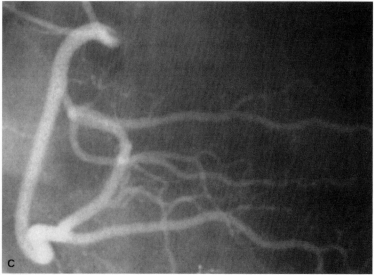

Figure 3-25. (A) Properly positioned cranial right anterior oblique (RAO) view of the right coronary artery (RCA) with inspiration. The posterior descending artery (PDA, *solid arrow*) and posterolateral branches (PLBs, *open arrows*) are nicely separated yet not projected over the diaphragm, and the posterolateral segment artery is projected in front of the body of the RCA. **(B)** With less RAO rotation (about 15 degrees), the crux *(arrowhead)* is adequately visualized, but the PDA and PLB are severely foreshortened. **(C)** Cranial RAO view with full exhalation results in projection of the distal branches over the diaphragm. Although there is adequate exposure in this instance, little diagnostic information has been gained at the expense of increased radiation exposure to the patient and increased scatter to the catheterization laboratory personnel.

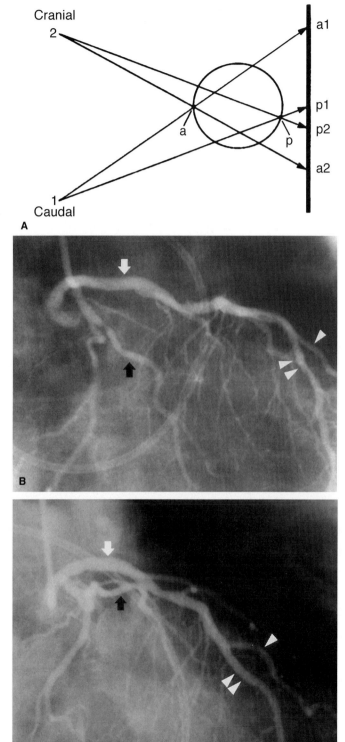

Figure 3-26. (A) Diagram showing changes in the projected positions of vessels on the anterior wall of the heart (e.g., acute marginals [a]), relative to those on the posterior wall (e.g., obtuse marginals [p]). With caudal angulation, anterior vessels are projected superior to the posterior branches (a1, p1); with cranial angulation, the posterior branches are projected superiorly (p2, a2). **(B)** Caudal and **(C)** cranial right anterior oblique views of the left coronary. Because the obtuse marginal *(black arrow)* is posterior relative to the left anterior descending (LAD) *(white arrow)*, it moves upward relative to the latter with cranial angulation. Likewise, the distal LAD *(double arrowheads)* moves down relative to the nearby diagonal *(single arrowhead)*.

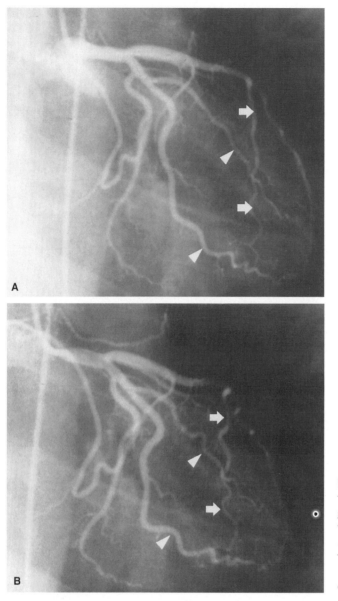

Figure 3-27. (A) Diastolic and **(B)** systolic frames from a left coronary arteriogram in the caudal right anterior oblique view. During systole, the obtuse marginal arteries *(arrowheads)* move upward toward the left anterior descending *(arrows)*. This is more evident when the coronary arteries are viewed in motion.

Cranial angulation causes the posterolateral branches to be projected superior to the PDA (Fig. 3-25*A*).The PLSA is also seen to better advantage because it is less foreshortened. This principle applies both when these vessels fill antegrade as well as when they fill by collaterals (see Fig. 3-19*B*) and is true regardless of coronary dominance. As with the straight RAO, moderation is important in setting up the Cr-RAO view of the RCA. As a rule, 25 to 30 degrees of RAO rotation and 20 to 25 degrees of cranial angulation yield the best results. Less tube rotation provides good visualization of the crux but foreshortens the PDA and posterolateral branches (Fig. 3-25*B*) and results in suboptimal x-ray factors. Too much rotation superimposes the distal RCA and PLSA and foreshortens the PDA and posterolateral branches, as it does in the RAO view (see Fig. 3-24*B*). Likewise, there is usually little to be gained by using extreme cranial angulation and having the patient exhale (Fig. 3-25*C*), because this technique severely foreshortens the body of the RCA and projects all the distal vessels over the diaphragm. The use of moderate angulation with a full inspiration usually separates the distal branches well and results in a picture of better quality.

Philosophy of Angiography of the Right Coronary Artery

In general, angiographic evaluation of the RCA is more straightforward than is that of the LCA because there are fewer branches to deal with. In most patients, a good study can be obtained with three views: lateral, Cr-LAO, and straight RAO. The Cr-RAO can be added as a fourth view if necessary, but it is not needed routinely because, as has been discussed, comparison of the Cr-LAO and RAO views indicates whether the Cr-RAO would be helpful. This is not the case with angiography of the LCA; in which the most important RAO view usually cannot be predicted. If the Cr-RAO view is preferred to the straight view, it is doubly important to not use an extreme view, such as that shown in Figure 3-25*C*. Finally, it is important not to end

up with three views of the RCA within a 50- to 60-degree arc (e.g., 40 degrees of LAO through 15 degrees of RAO rotation); this violates the rule of trying to obtain orthogonal views. Although it is difficult to say with certainty, in a very unstable patient, the two most important views are probably either the lateral and Cr-RAO or the Cr-LAO and Cr-RAO views.

Other Considerations

The way vessels move in relation to each other on the Cd-RAO and Cr-RAO views can help the angiographer identify them if they fill by collaterals and their origins are not apparent. Because the acute marginals are on the anterior wall of the heart and the obtuse marginals are on the posterior wall, caudal and cranial angulations cause them to move in opposite directions (Fig. 3-26). The general rule is that caudal angulation throws posterior vessels inferiorly. All the other projectional movements can be derived from this rule: posterior vessels move upward with cranial angulation, anterior vessels move downward with cranial angulation, and anterior vessels move upward with caudal angulation. It is therefore a simple matter to determine the location of a collaterally filled vessel by noticing which way it moves with caudal or cranial angulation. The same applies to the PDA relative to the posterolateral branches. Because the PDA is anterior relative to the posterolateral branches, it moves upward with caudal angulation and the posterolateral branches move downward. This observation may be important if the PDA is obstructed at its origin.

Another common problem involves differentiation of the LAD from a diagonal when one or both of them fill from collaterals. Watching the way in which the suspect vessel moves can usually answer this question. Diagonal and obtuse marginal arteries tend to move concordantly because both are on the lateral wall of the heart; the LAD, being relatively anterior, moves discordantly when compared with the obtuse marginal arteries (Fig. 3-27). This phenomenon can be especially helpful if a lateral view is not available or if both the LAD and the diagonal are occluded.

REFERENCES

1. McAlpine WA. Heart and coronary arteries. New York: Springer-Verlag, 1975:134.
2. Meyerovitz MF, Reagan K, Friedman PL. Caudal-posteroanterior view in coronary arteriography. Radiology 1989;171:866.
3. Bunnell IL, Greene DG, Tandon RN, et al. The half axial projection: a new look at the proximal left coronary artery. Circulation 1973;48:1151.
4. Elliott LP, Bream PR, Soto B, et al. The significance of the caudal-left anterior oblique view in analyzing the left main coronary artery and its major branches. Radiology 1981;139:39.
5. Green CE, Elliott LP, Rogers WJ, et al. The importance of angled right anterior oblique views in improving visualization of the coronary arteries. Part II: craniocaudal view. Radiology 1982;142:637.
6. Elliott LP, Green CE, Rogers WJ, et al. The importance of angled right anterior oblique views in improving visualization of the coronary arteries. Part I: caudocranial view. Radiology 1982;142:631.

Coronary Cinematography, by Curtis E. Green.
Lippincott–Raven Publishers, © 1995.

CHAPTER *FOUR*

Abnormalities of the Coronary Arteries

Atherosclerosis accounts for the vast majority of problems encountered in the coronary circulation; however, there are several other entities that can result in clinically significant disease. These include embolism, spasm, myocardial bridging, inflammatory diseases, aneurysms, and dissection. Coronary arteriography, despite its limitations, remains the only way to definitively evaluate coronary anatomy. The significance of a given lesion or series of lesions may be difficult to ascertain in many circumstances, requiring functional tests such as radionuclide studies for clarification.

CORONARY ATHEROSCLEROSIS

The most common and important abnormality of the coronary arteries is atherosclerotic narrowing, and known or suspected coronary artery disease is the most frequent indication for cardiac catheterization. Angiographic diagnosis of coronary atherosclerosis is based on identification of any of the following: focal or diffuse narrowing that persists after intracoronary administration of nitroglycerin, irregularity without measurable narrowing, or ectasia. In most cases, more than one of these is present. Interpretations of coronary angiograms should describe lesion location, severity, length, and morphology.

69

Discrete Stenosis

The most common angiographic pattern observed is that of one or more discrete stenoses. These stenoses are discrete only in a relative sense, because there is usually some degree of generalized narrowing of the remainder of the vessel.[1] The severity of luminal narrowing is fairly easy to determine in this circumstance, because the adjacent vessel has a relatively normal appearance (Fig. 4-1). This assumption may lure the angiographer into a false sense of security about the severity of the stenosis, however (Fig. 4-2). The various ways to measure coronary narrowing are discussed in Chapter 5.

Coronary stenoses appear to be more common in the proximal portions of the epicardial vessels and at vessel bifurcations (Fig. 4-3), perhaps

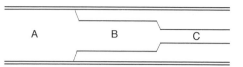

Figure 4-2. The problem with estimating the severity of stenosis when diffuse narrowing is present. If normal vessel luminal diameter is at region A, then narrowing in region B would be graded as 50% stenosis and that in region C as 75% stenosis. If the entire vessel is narrowed to the extent present in region B, however, region C will appear to be narrowed only 50%, and the severity of narrowing will be underestimated.

because of turbulent flow in the latter case. These stenoses can be classified both pathologically and angiographically as either "simple" or "complex."[2] *Simple stenoses* consist of fibrous or fatty plaques with intact luminal surfaces and have a fairly low likelihood of causing unstable angina or acute myocardial infarction. On angiograms, they appear to have smooth lumens without any evidence of undermining or filling defects (see Fig. 4-1), and they can be either

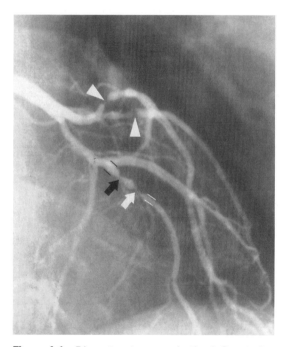

Figure 4-1. Discrete stenoses in the left anterior descending and first diagonal branch *(arrowheads)* and sequential stenoses in the inferior branch of the first obtuse marginal *(arrows)*. Choosing the reference diameter for the marginal lesions is more difficult because the vessel tapers significantly over a short distance. Percent stenosis will be higher if the *black lines* are chosen and lower if the *white lines* are used.

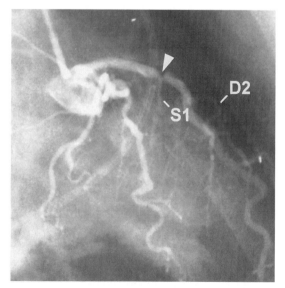

Figure 4-3. Stenosis of the proximal left anterior descending *(arrowhead)* at the first septal (S1). (D2, second diagonal.)

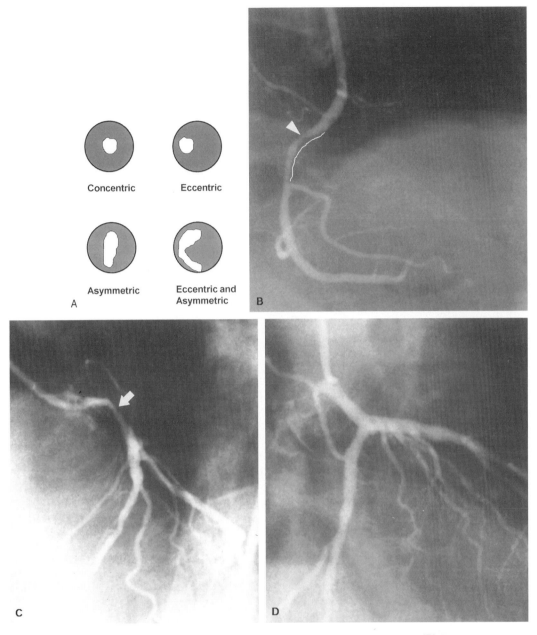

Figure 4-4. Simple lesions. **(A)** Diagram of different stenosis morphologies. **(B)** Eccentric stenosis of the mid right coronary *(arrowhead)*. The *white line* delineates the expected course of the wall of the vessel. **(C)** Cranial left anterior oblique (LAO) and **(D)** right anterior oblique views of the left coronary showing an asymmetric stenosis of the left main *(arrow)*. The stenosis is centrally located and thus concentric but is apparent only in the cranial LAO view.

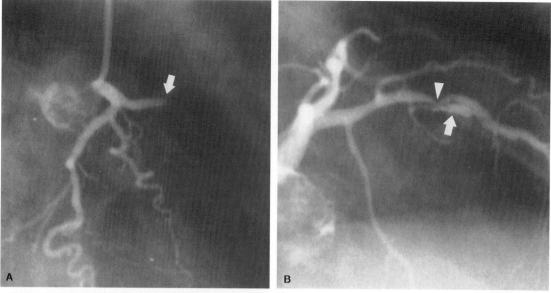

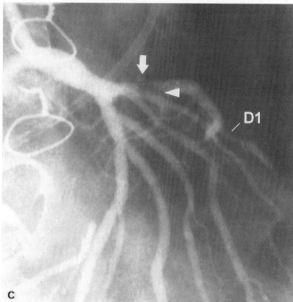

Figure 4-5. Complex lesions. **(A)** Thrombotic occlusion of the proximal left anterior descending (LAD; *arrow*). **(B)** Huge ulcerated plaque *(arrow)* in the mid LAD, beginning at a high-grade stenosis *(arrowhead)*. **(C)** Small ulceration *(arrow)* in the proximal LAD just before the origin of the first septal *(arrowhead)*. (D1, first diagonal.)

concentric or eccentric (Fig. 4-4). *Complex lesions* are characterized by plaque rupture, intraplaque hemorrhage, or thrombosis and are strongly associated with acute ischemic syndromes.[2] Angiographically, these are characterized by one or more of the following features: irregular or hazy edges, ulceration, filling defects, and undermining (Fig. 4-5). Compared with postmortem examination and coronary an-

gioscopy, angiography has been shown to be insensitive but fairly specific for identification of complex lesions.[2] Intravascular ultrasound has confirmed this assessment.[3]

Coronary occlusions can result from gradually increasing atherosclerotic plaque, acute thrombosis after plaque rupture, or coronary embolism. The first of these tends to cause a tapered-appearing occlusion Fig. 4-6), and the latter two

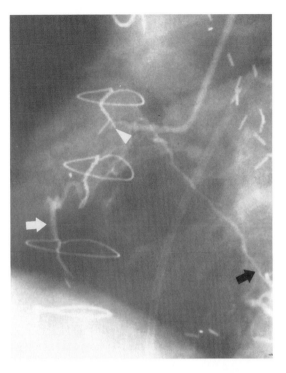

Figure 4-6. Chronic occlusion of the right coronary artery (RCA; *arrowhead)* with collaterals to the distal RCA *(white arrow)* and to the posterolateral segment artery via a Kugel collateral *(black arrow).*

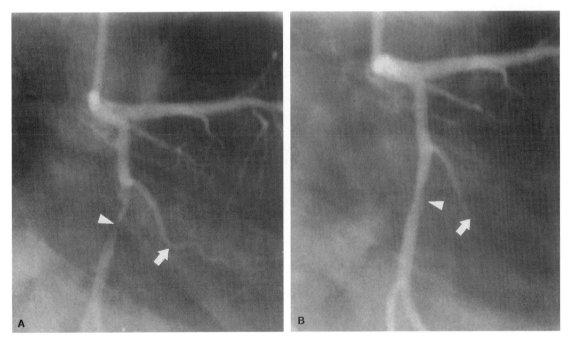

Figure 4-7. Embolic occlusion of the second obtuse marginal after balloon dilatation of the distal left circumflex. **(A)** Before angioplasty, the second marginal (M2) is angiographically normal *(arrow).* The stenosis *(arrowhead)* does not involve the origin of M2. **(B)** After angioplasty, there is abrupt occlusion of M2 *(arrow),* with only a small dissection at the dilatation site *(arrowhead),* which does not appear to extend back to the origin of M2.

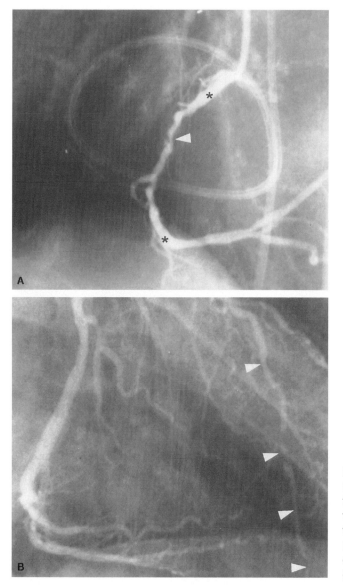

Figure 4-8. (A) Diffuse narrowing of the right coronary artery (RCA). Although there is a relatively discrete stenosis in the mid RCA *(arrowhead)*, most of the vessel is narrowed to some degree *(between asterisks)*. **(B)** Diffuse narrowing of the distal left anterior descending *(arrowheads)* with multiple stenoses.

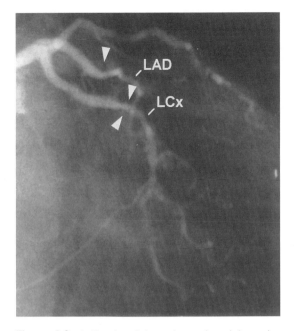

Figure 4-9. Intimal calcium *(arrowheads)* marks the true diameters of the left anterior descending (LAD) and left circumflex (LCx) arteries.

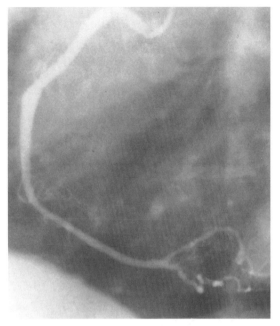

Figure 4-10. Gradual tapering of the distal right coronary artery (RCA) makes selection of a reference diameter difficult distally. There may also be mild ectasia in the mid RCA.

usually cause abrupt termination of the vessel. Embolic occlusions are characterized by a margin that is convex proximally (Fig. 4-7) but are in reality usually suggested only if the coronary arteries otherwise appear relatively normal and the patient has a problem that predisposes to emboli.

Diffuse Disease

Pathologically, coronary artery disease is a diffuse process with localized exacerbations. Angiographically, the localized regions are recognized as stenoses, with the remainder of the vessel appearing normal. In many patients, however, there are long areas of angiographically apparent narrowing (Fig. 4-8) which can be characterized either as long, focal stenoses or perhaps more accurately, as localized areas of diffuse narrowing. These can be recognized in a number of ways. Recognition is easiest when the vessel on both ends of the stenosis is significantly greater in caliber than the suspect region. Cal-

cium in the vessel wall that is clearly seen to be outside the visualized lumen can also give a clue (Fig. 4-9). Vessels that gradually narrow are the most difficult to characterize (Fig. 4-10). It may be impossible to tell normal tapering from diffuse narrowing, especially if a major branch vessel comes off just before the vessel begins to taper.

In some patients, narrowing is so diffuse and severe that individual stenoses cannot be confidently measured (Fig. 4-11). Irregular vessels that appear to be considerably smaller than would be expected for a given patient may provide a clue to this situation. In these cases, any stenosis measurement is likely to be grossly inaccurate, so it is probably better to state that the entire segment or vessel is diffusely narrowed and try to estimate whether the narrowing is more or less than whatever is considered significant (e.g., diffuse up to 90%, diffuse 50% to 75%, diffuse less than 50%). Keep in mind that, although it is less important than cross-sectional area, stenosis length also determines resistance to flow.

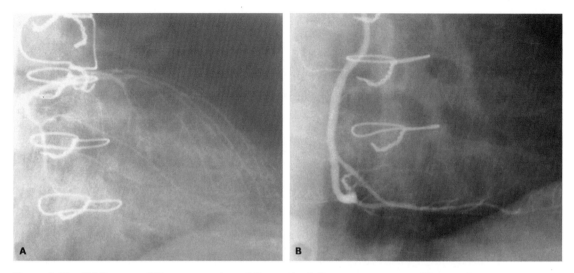

Figure 4-11. (A) Severe, diffuse narrowing of the entire left coronary artery. All vessels appear very small, but no discrete stenoses can be seen. **(B)** The right coronary artery appears relatively normal.

Coronary Thrombus

Clot is frequently seen in both unstable angina[4] and acute myocardial infarction.[5,6] Angiographic diagnosis of thrombus in the coronary arteries is made difficult by several factors, including limited resolution and poor vessel filling distal to severe stenoses. Clots can appear as filling defects within the lumen or, in the case of thrombotic occlusion, as abrupt vessel cutoff, sometimes with staining by contrast (Fig. 4-12). Before assuming that a filling defect represents thrombus, the cineangiographer should be careful to exclude other causes of filling defects. These include flow artifacts from poor filling (Fig. 4-13) and collateral flow (Fig. 4-14). Clot should not come and go with the phases of the cardiac cycle, and any filling defect that does so is more likely to be caused by streaming or unopacified blood from collaterals.

Coronary Ectasia

Ectasia of the coronary arteries can cause either localized aneurysm formation or diffuse dilatation. Severe, diffuse coronary ectasia (Fig. 4-15A) is uncommon but can be associated with significant symptoms and, in some cases, has a prognosis similar to that of medically treated triple vessel disease, even in the absence of coronary obstruction.[7] This is probably related to the propensity of ectatic coronary arteries to harbor thrombus (Fig. 4-15B). More common is localized ectasia. Angiographically, this can appear either as dilatation and irregularity over a short segment of coronary artery (Fig. 4-16A) or as a discrete aneurysm, frequently at a vessel bifurcation (Fig. 4-16B). Localized ectasia can cause significant problems for the angiographer because it effectively removes any normal reference vessel to which a lesion can be compared (Fig. 4-17). Discrete aneurysms can obscure vessel bifurcations and make evaluation of the origins of side branches difficult (see Fig. 4-16B).

An important cause of coronary aneurysm in children is mucocutaneous lymph node syndrome, also known as Kawasaki disease,[8] which causes a vasculitis involving the walls of the coronary arteries and results in focal destructive lesions. Both saccular and cylindrical aneurysms can be formed, and they are frequently interspersed with areas of focal narrowing that result

(text continues on p. 81)

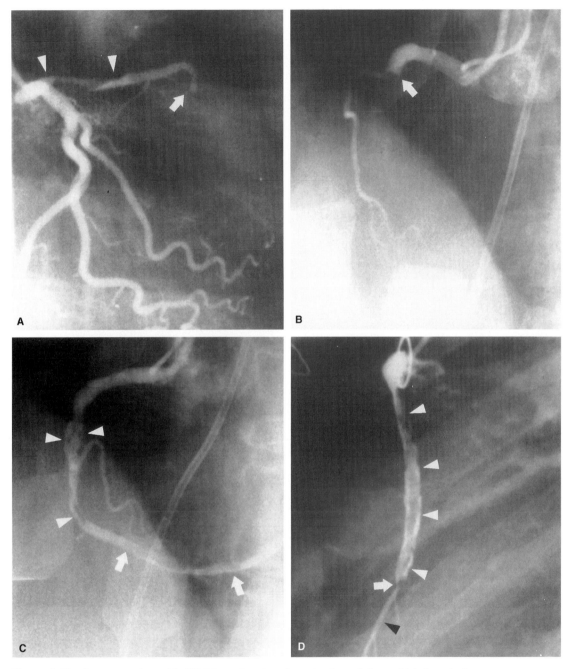

Figure 4-12. Coronary thrombi. **(A)** There is abrupt occlusion of the mid left anterior descending *(arrow)* as well as a long filling defect proximally *(arrowheads)*. **(B)** Abrupt occlusion of the proximal right coronary with a concave margin *(arrow)*. A coronary embolus could have a similar appearance. **(C)** Extensive clot after acute myocardial infarction with thrombolytic therapy. There are small, linear filling defects in the mid vessel *(arrowheads)* and a very long defect distally *(between arrows)*. **(D)** Saphenous vein graft to the left anterior descending (*black arrowhead*) with extensive thrombus *(white arrowheads)* and a severe stenosis at the distal anastomosis *(arrow)*.

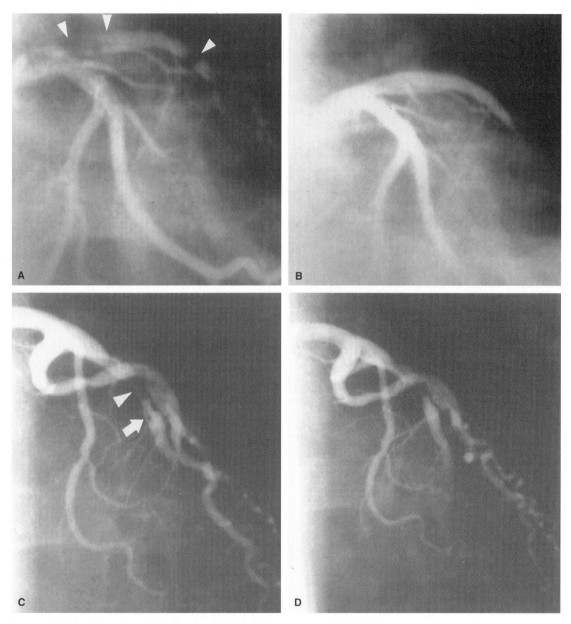

Figure 4-13. Streaming artifacts that simulate thrombus. **(A, B)** Right anterior oblique (RAO) views of the left coronary artery (LCA). There are large filling defects in the left anterior descending (LAD; *arrowheads)* that disappear with better filling of the vessel. These were interpreted as thrombus. **(C, D)** RAO views of the LCA in a different patient with a high-grade mid LAD stenosis *(arrowhead)*. The small, linear filling defect distal to the stenosis *(arrow)* disappears on the later frame.

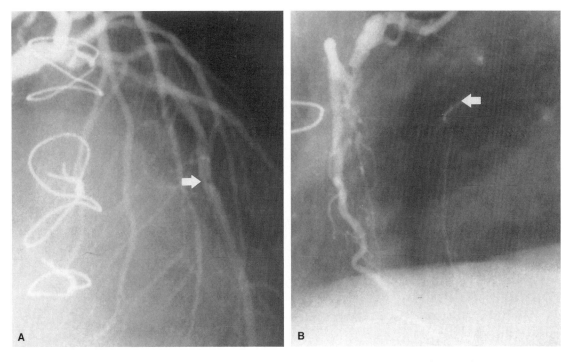

Figure 4-14. Collateral flow artifact. **(A)** Cranial right anterior oblique view of the left coronary. A small filling defect is seen in the mid anterior descending (*arrow*). **(B)** Lateral view of the right coronary artery demonstrates a collateral to the mid anterior descending from the posterior descending, which enters at the site of the filling defect (*arrow*).

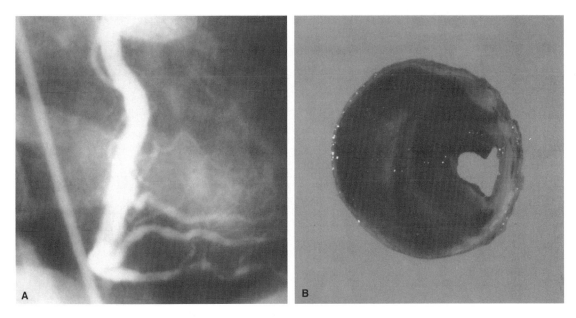

Figure 4-15. **(A)** Ectasia involving the entire body of the right coronary artery. **(B)** Pathology specimen of an ectatic coronary artery from another patient. Most of the lumen is filled with thrombus.

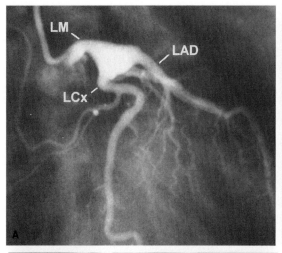

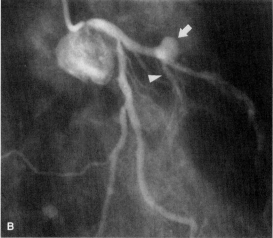

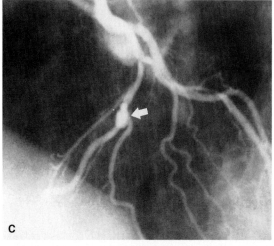

Figure 4-16. (A) Ectasia of the left main (LM) extending into the left anterior descending (LAD) and left circumflex (LCx). **(B)** Discrete aneurysm of the LAD *(arrow)* arising at the origin of the first septal perforator *(arrowhead)*. **(C)** Discrete LAD aneurysm at the origin of the second diagonal *(arrow)*.

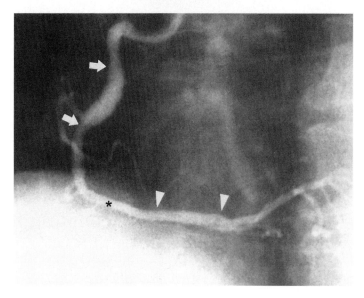

Figure 4-17. There is a long area of mild to moderate ectasia *(arrows)* in the proximal right coronary artery (RCA), followed by an area of narrower but smooth vessel *(asterisk)*. Distally, the RCA dilates again *(arrowheads)*.

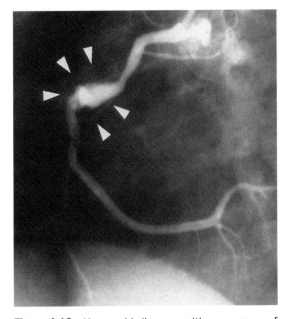

Figure 4-18. Kawasaki disease with aneurysm of the mid right coronary artery. Calcium in the wall *(arrowheads)* marks the true size of the clot-filled aneurysm.

from scar formation. Proximal portions of the coronary arteries are often involved (Fig. 4-18). Complications caused by involvement of the coronaries can occur as early as the first week of the disease or as late as 16 years later. These complications include both acute thrombosis and chronic ischemia from constriction. Most aneurysms begin to resolve within 6 to 12 months.

Other causes of coronary dilatation include polyarteritis nodosa, scleroderma, syphilis, Ehlers-Danlos syndrome, bacterial infection, and congenital dilatation. These conditions are generally differentiated from atherosclerotic aneurysms by the clinical presentation rather than by angiographic findings. Syphilis more typically causes coronary ostial stenosis; about a quarter of patients with syphilitic aortitis have coronary ostial involvement.[9]

CORONARY ARTERY SPASM

Pure coronary artery spasm is a less common cause of myocardial ischemia than is atheroscle-

rosis, but it may contribute to ischemia in patients with underlying coronary narrowing.[10] Coronary spasm is classically associated with variant (Prinzmetal) angina, but angiographically there are three circumstances in which spasm is seen: at the tip of the catheter (Fig. 4-19), spontaneously in patients with or without other coronary stenoses (Fig. 4-20), and after administration of ergonovine or acetylcholine in patients with Prinzmetal angina (Fig. 4-21). Catheter-induced spasm is more common in the right coronary artery (RCA) but can occur in other vessels, including the left main. Because of the possibility of secondary vasoconstriction with any stenosis, it is an excellent policy to routinely give intracoronary nitroglycerin to any patient with coronary narrowing. This is true no matter how typically atherosclerotic a lesion appears. The usual dose is 120 μg to 180 μg. Sublingual and intravenous nitroglycerin do not as reliably result in coronary dilatation and relief of spasm.

Ergonovine stimulation is used if there is a suspicion of coronary spasm and the coronary arteries have no significant fixed narrowing. It can be given either by intraarterial (not intracoronary) administration or intravenously. There are many protocols for ergonovine testing, but all are variations on a progressive dose system that begins with a low dose, such as 0.05 mg, and gradually increases the dose until a total of 0.40 mg has been given (e.g., 0.05 mg, 0.10 mg, and 0.25 mg). Some angiographers prefer to film the coronaries after each dose; others take pictures only after the last dose unless the patient develops chest pain or electrocardiographic changes. If spasm occurs, it is usually relieved by sublingual nitroglycerin or nifedipine; occasionally, intracoronary nitroglycerin is required. For this reason, and because some significant spasm can be clinically silent, it is inadvisable to perform ergonovine testing outside of the catheterization laboratory. Ergonovine-induced vasospasm can be either focal or diffuse (see Fig. 4-21*A*, *B*). The normal response to ergonovine is a mild, diffuse diminution in caliber of the coronary arteries.

Acetylcholine appears to selectively cause vasoconstriction in vessels with abnormal endothe-

(text continues on p. 84)

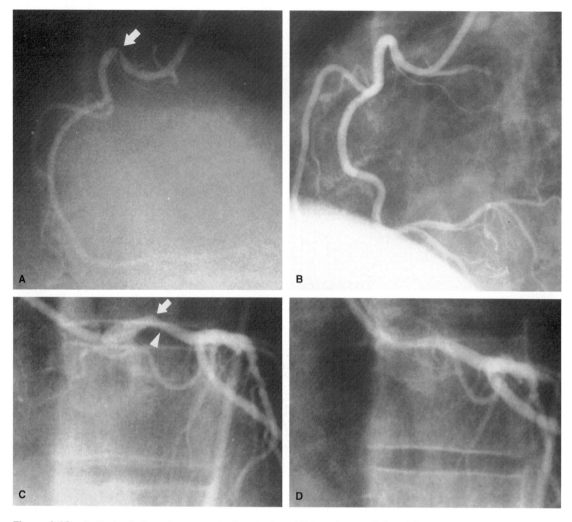

Figure 4-19. Catheter-induced spasm. Left anterior oblique views of the right coronary artery **(A)** before and **(B)** after intracoronary administration of nitroglycerin. Spasm occurred at the catheter tip *(arrow)*. **(C)** Shallow left anterior oblique view of the left coronary artery shows moderate narrowing of the left main *(arrowhead)* just distal to the catheter tip *(arrow)*. **(D)** Narrowing disappears after intracoronary administration of nitroglycerin.

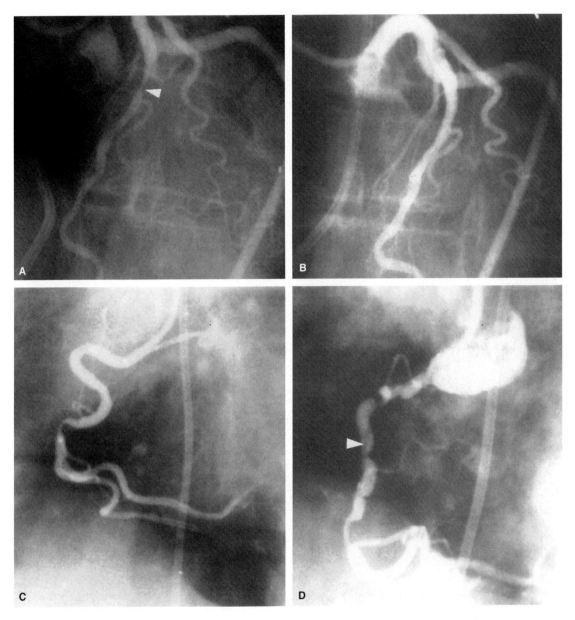

Figure 4-20. Spontaneous spasm. Views of the left coronary artery **(A)** before and **(B)** after nitroglycerin administration showing spasm just proximal to the second diagonal *(arrowhead)*. **(C–E)** Spasm related to attempted coronary angioplasty. **(C)** Before dilatation, there is a significant stenosis in the mid right coronary artery with an otherwise unremarkable vessel. **(D)** After balloon dilatation, numerous stenoses are present proximal to the dilatation site, and a small intimal flap is present *(arrowhead)*. *(continued)*

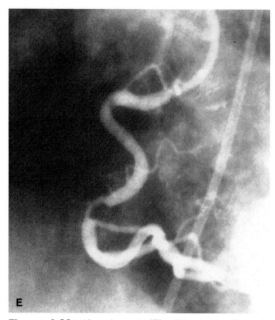

Figure 4-20. *(Continued)* **(E)** After nitroglycerin without further dilatation, the new stenoses have disappeared.

lial function, such as occurs with atherosclerosis.[11] If spasm is induced, the angiographic findings are similar to those seen after ergonovine administration (see Fig. 4-21C).

MYOCARDIAL BRIDGES

Occasionally, a coronary artery travels in the myocardium instead of on the epicardial surface, resulting in systolic compression of the artery. The left anterior descending (LAD) artery is the most commonly involved vessel (Fig. 4-22), but diagonal and obtuse marginal branches are occasionally affected. Muscle bridges in the distal RCA are rare and may cause a kinking appearance of the vessel rather than typical compression (Fig. 4-23). Other vessels are rarely involved. Systolic compression is also frequently seen in patients with hypertrophic cardiomyopathy (Fig. 4-24). Although LAD muscle bridges are usually benign,[12] some patients with otherwise normal coronary arteries have had exertional angina associated with a muscle bridge,

which was relieved by operative decompression of the coronary artery. Confirmation of myocardial ischemia by physiologic testing should be done before operative therapy is considered.

COLLATERAL BLOOD FLOW

One of the reasons that patients with coronary artery disease present with such a variety of symptoms is the marked variability in collateral blood flow to obstructed vessels. There is a plethora of potential collateral pathways that may develop in the presence of obstruction. Some are present before any obstruction, as evidenced by immediate collateral filling of vessels obstructed by spasm; others develop after a period of gradually increasing obstruction or in the aftermath of an acute occlusion.

Some of the confusion caused by the angiographic appearance of collaterals can be diminished by remembering that for one vessel to supply blood to another, the vessels must have some common ground; that is, they must be joined by a piece of myocardium. Collaterals do not wander through chambers! Accordingly, collaterals may develop over the epicardial surface, in the myocardium, or through the atrial or ventricular septae.

Intracoronary collaterals allow filling of the distal portion of an occluded vessel from the proximal portion of the same vessel. They can be recognized by their tortuous course outside the normal path of the involved coronary artery (Fig. 4-25). It is often difficult to distinguish between filling through intracoronary collaterals and subtotal occlusion with antegrade flow.

Intercoronary collaterals exist either between different coronary arteries (contralateral collaterals) or between branches of the same coronary artery (ipsilateral collaterals). In rare instances, collaterals to the coronary arteries come from the bronchial or pericardial arteries.[13]

Although collaterals are more likely to be present if there is complete obstruction of a vessel, they may also occur in the presence of

(text continues on p. 88)

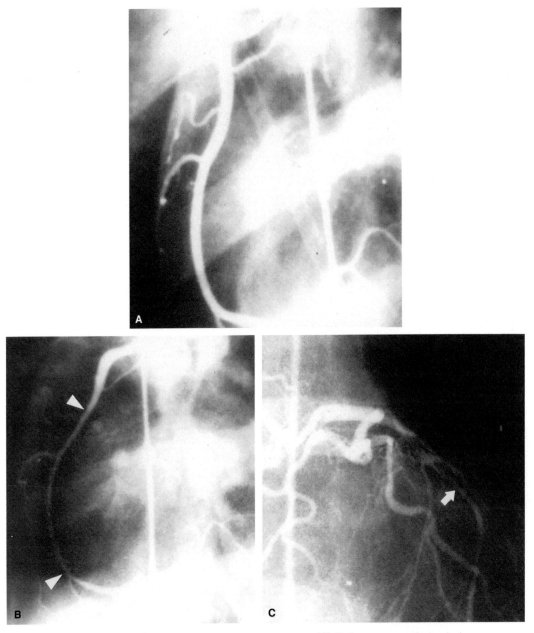

Figure 4-21. Pharmacologically induced coronary spasm. **(A)** Before ergonovine admin-istration, the right coronary artery is angiographically normal. **(B)** After administration of ergonovine, there is severe, diffuse narrowing of the entire mid vessel *(arrowheads)*. **(C)** Increased narrowing in the mid left anterior descending *(arrow)* after administration of acetylcholine in a patient with coronary artery disease.

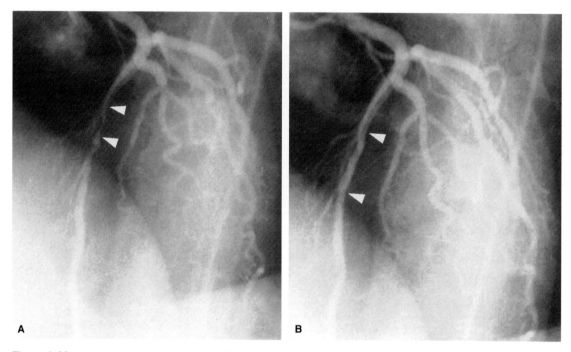

Figure 4-22. Left anterior descending (LAD) muscle bridge. **(A)** Systolic and **(B)** diastolic frames show compression of the LAD *(arrowheads)* during systole without residual narrowing during diastole.

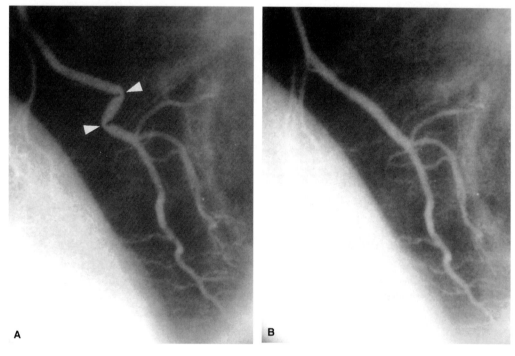

Figure 4-23. Right coronary artery (RCA) muscle bridge. **(A)** During systole, there is kinking of the distal RCA *(arrowheads)*. **(B)** No kinking is seen during diastole. At operation, the RCA was found to be intramyocardial in this location.

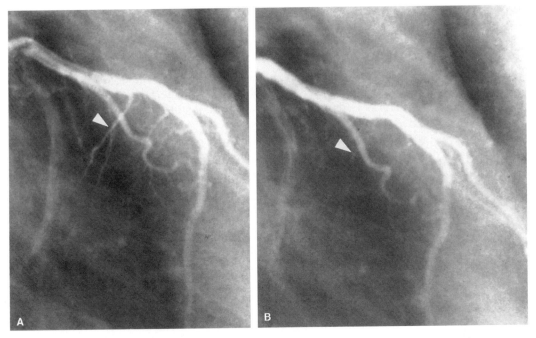

Figure 4-24. Septal compression in hypertrophic cardiomyopathy. Septal branch *(arrowhead)* present during diastole **(A)** almost disappears during systole **(B)**.

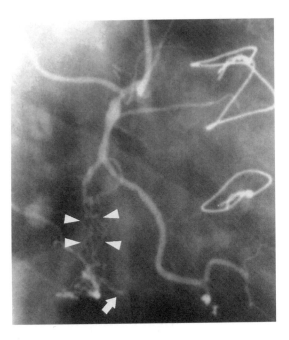

Figure 4-25. Intracoronary collaterals *(arrowheads)* fill the distal branches of the right coronary artery *(arrow)*.

subtotal occlusion, and they occasionally occur in the presence of apparently moderate coronary narrowing. Collaterals to a vessel may also be present from more than one source. If this occurs, the vessel caught between the two collateral sources may be poorly opacified because of the competitive flow. The cineangiographer may then be tempted to conclude that there is significant disease in the vessel when there may in fact be none. A typical instance of this occurs in the posterolateral segment artery (PLSA) when the posterior descending artery (PDA) fills through the ventricular septum and the posterolateral branches fill through the left atrioventricular groove from the left circumflex.

Collaterals to the Right Coronary Artery

Ipsilateral Collaterals

The RCA can supply collaterals to itself through the anterior right ventricular (RV) free wall, through the atrial or ventricular septum, or on the right atrial wall. One of the most common

pathways between the distal and the proximal portions of the RCA uses anterior wall vessels such as the conus artery or an early acute marginal artery to supply either a more distal acute marginal artery or the PDA at the apex (Fig. 4-26). These can be recognized on right anterior oblique views by their course on the ventricular side of the atrioventricular groove (to the right of the RCA when looking at the film). Another important collateral pathway is from the sinoatrial node artery to the atrioventricular node artery through the atrial septum (Kugel's collateral; Fig. 4-27). Less common collateral pathways include atrial branches of the RCA and collaterals from a right superior septal perforator to the PDA through the ventricular septum (Fig. 4-28). One interesting, roundabout collateral pathway is from the conus artery to an occluded LAD (circle of Vieussens), which then fills the PDA through septal collaterals.

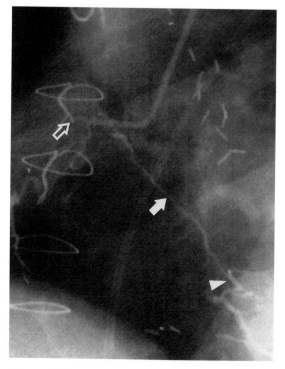

Figure 4-27. Kugel's collateral. Atrial collateral *(solid arrow)* arising proximal to the right coronary artery (RCA) occlusion *(open arrow)* fills the distal RCA through the atrioventricular node artery *(arrowhead)*.

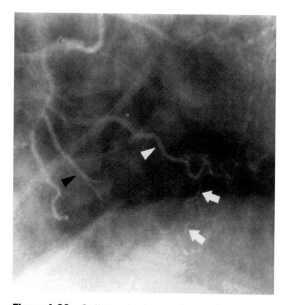

Figure 4-26. Collaterals *(arrows)* over the anterior wall of the right ventricle connect two marginal branches *(black and white arrowheads)*.

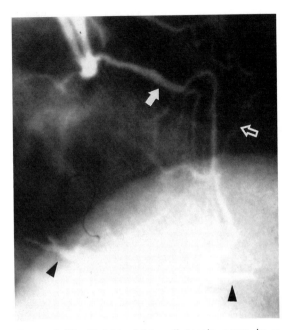

Figure 4-28. Right-to-right collaterals seen in a cranial right anterior oblique view. The right superior septal perforator *(solid arrow)* supplies the posterior descending *(arrowheads)* through the ventricular septum. There is also a collateral from a proximal acute marginal to a more distal one *(open arrow)*.

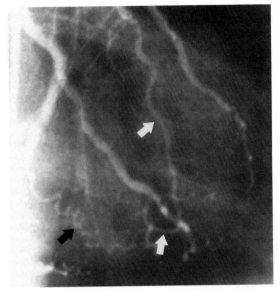

Figure 4-29. Collateral from the left anterior descending *(white arrows)* to an acute marginal *(black arrow)*.

Contralateral Collaterals

The left coronary artery (LCA) can supply collaterals to the RCA by several pathways: anterior RV wall, posterior left ventricular (LV) wall, ventricular septum, left atrioventricular groove, left atrium and atrial septum, and around the apex. The LAD commonly supplies the RCA either through RV branches of the LAD that connect to acute marginals (Fig. 4-29), around the apex directly to the distal PDA (Fig. 4-30*A*), or through septal perforators (Figure 4-30*B*). Less common collaterals include LAD to conus artery and LAD to a long posterolateral branch that extends to the LV apex.

The most common collaterals from the circumflex system to the RCA are those from obtuse marginals to posterolateral branches (Fig. 4-31) and atrioventricular groove collaterals from the distal circumflex to the PLSA (Fig. 4-32). Atrial septal collaterals to the atrioventric-

ular node artery also occur, resulting in what can be loosely termed a left Kugel's artery.

Other collateral pathways are possible; however, connections such as acute marginal to diagonal, acute marginal to obtuse marginal, or septal perforator to posterolateral branch would not be expected, because these regions are not in physical continuity. Also keep in mind that the same collateral pathways occur in both left dominant and codominant systems.

Collaterals to the Left Coronary Artery

Ipsilateral Collaterals

LCA-to-LCA collaterals occur over the LV free wall, through the ventricular septum, and in the atrioventricular groove. Proximal to distal LAD collaterals usually involve flow from a proximal

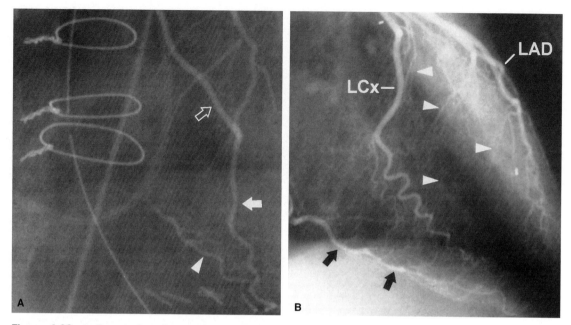

Figure 4-30. Left anterior descending (LAD) to posterior descending artery (PDA) collaterals. **(A)** The LAD *(solid arrow)* supplies the PDA *(arrowhead)* at the apex. The LAD is filling from a coronary bypass graft *(open arrow)* in this patient. **(B)** The PDA *(arrows)* is filling from the LAD through numerous septal perforators *(arrowheads)*. (LCx, left circumflex.)

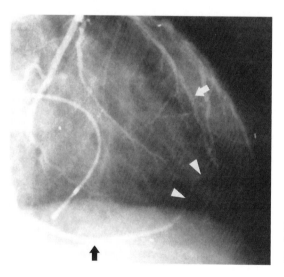

Figure 4-31. Collateral *(arrowheads)* from an obtuse marginal *(white arrow)* to a posterolateral branch of the right coronary *(black arrow)*.

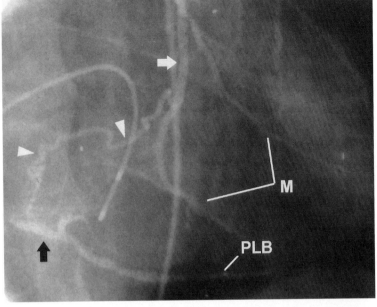

Figure 4-32. Left atrioventricular groove collateral *(arrowheads)* from the distal left circumflex *(white arrow)* to the posterolateral segment artery *(black arrow).* (M, obtuse marginals; PLB, posterolateral branch.)

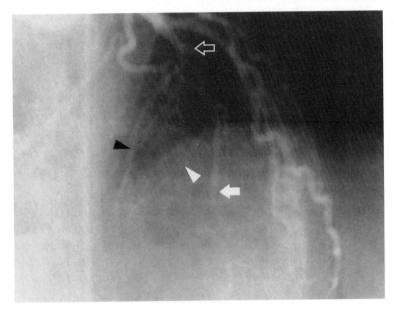

Figure 4-33. Septal collaterals *(black and white arrowheads)* fill the left anterior descending *(solid arrow)* distal to the occlusion site *(open arrow).*

diagonal to either a distal diagonal or the distal LAD. Another common pathway is through the ventricular septum from a proximal septal perforator to a more distal one (Fig. 4-33). The main pathways for collaterals to the left circumflex are the atrioventricular groove and the lateral LV wall. The latter can provide diagonal to marginal, marginal to marginal, or LAD to marginal connections (Fig. 4-34).

Contralateral Collaterals

Collaterals from the RCA to the LCA use the same pathways described for LCA-to-RCA col-

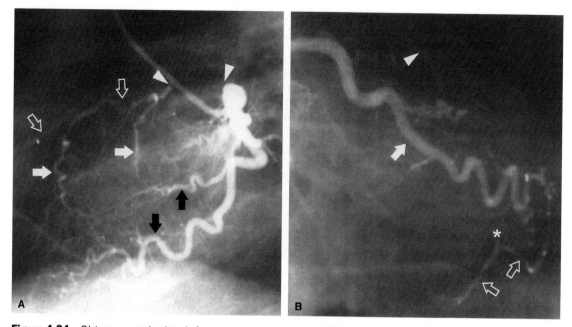

Figure 4-34. Obtuse marginal to left anterior descending (LAD) collaterals. **(A)** The LAD is occluded proximally *(between arrowheads)*. The mid LAD *(open arrows)* fills from diagonals *(white arrows)*, which have filled from obtuse marginals *(black arrows)*. **(B)** A large obtuse marginal *(solid arrow)* directly fills the terminal branches of the LAD *(open arrows)* back to its bifurcation *(asterisk)*. Faint filling of a diagonal is also seen *(arrowhead)*.

laterals (Fig. 4-35). These include the left atrioventricular groove (PLSA to distal circumflex), lateral LV wall (posterolateral branches to obtuse marginals or diagonals), anterior RV wall (acute marginals or conus to LAD), ventricular septum (septal perforator to septal perforator), and apex (PDA to LAD).

EVALUATION OF CORONARY ARTERY BYPASS GRAFTS

Because coronary atherosclerosis is a progressive disease, many patients who undergo coronary bypass eventually have recurrent symptoms and need repeat angiography. In some, the return of symptoms results from progression of disease in the native circulation; in others, there is obstruction of the bypass grafts. Long-term patency of venous grafts is determined by several factors, including atherogenic factors in the patient,

systemic blood pressure, surgical technique, and runoff into the bypassed vessel. If symptoms recur shortly after surgery, the cause is often occlusion of a graft. Late recurrence may be caused by graft occlusion, graft stenosis, or progression of disease in the native vessels. Occasionally, a graft is inadvertently placed proximal to the site of obstruction or into a coronary vein.

The majority of coronary bypass grafts are done with saphenous veins, but the left internal mammary artery (LIMA) has in many centers become the graft of choice for bypass of the LAD and can also be placed to a diagonal. There is good evidence that the LIMA is superior to vein grafts with regard to long-term patency.[14] Less frequently used as grafts are the right internal mammary artery (RIMA), either intact or as a free graft, the cephalic vein, and the gastroepiploic artery. Cannulization of the gastroepiploic artery can provide a challenge to the angiographer who does not have experience with abdominal angiography.

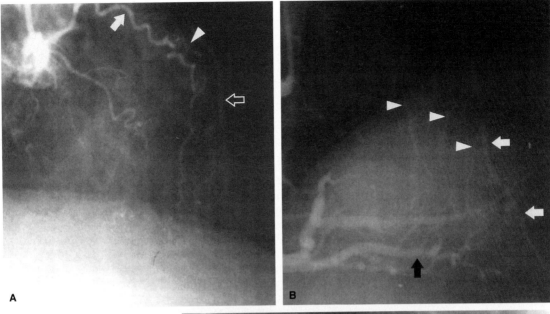

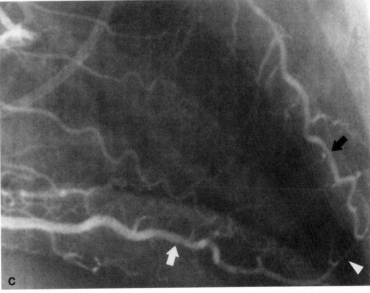

Figure 4-35. Right coronary to left anterior descending (LAD) collaterals. **(A)** Small collateral vessel *(arrowhead)* connects the conus artery *(solid arrow)* to the LAD *(open arrow)*. **(B)** Septal collaterals *(arrowheads)* from the posterior descending artery (PDA, *black arrow*) to the LAD *(white arrows)*. **(C)** Apical collateral *(arrowhead)* from the PDA *(white arrow)* to the LAD *(black arrow)*.

Saphenous Vein Grafts

Angiographic study of saphenous vein grafts is facilitated by marking the graft orifices with a radiopaque ring at the time of operation. Unfortunately, some surgeons are reluctant to do this, citing a variety of reasons from inconvenience to inflammation. If the graft orifices are not marked, it is crucial that the angiographer

know how many grafts were placed and, preferably, where they were placed. If there is any doubt about the number and status of the grafts, ascending aortography should be performed.

With Judkins' technique, most grafts can be cannulated with either a right bypass graft catheter or a right Judkins catheter. These are similar in appearance; however, the tip of the bypass catheter is slightly less curved. In a minority of

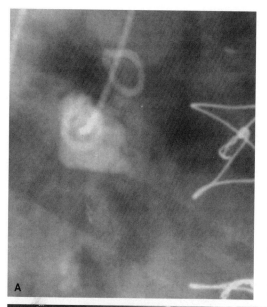

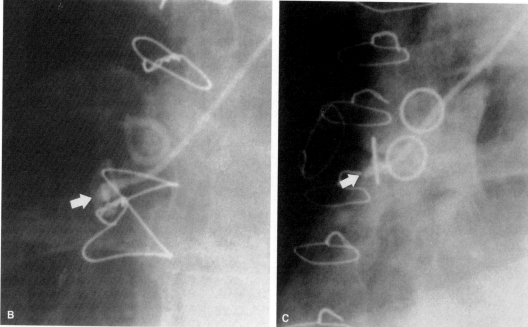

Figure 4-36. Bypass graft occlusions at proximal anastomosis. **(A)** In the right anterior oblique view, the graft stump is not visualized and the catheter could be pointed directly away from the graft. **(B)** Rotation to the frontal projection shows the stump of the graft projecting beyond the marker ring *(arrow).* **(C)** In a second patient, the ring is completely profiled and readily demonstrates the occluded graft *(arrow).*

cases, a left bypass catheter or other catheter is necessary.

The same principles that apply to angiography of the native coronary arteries apply to graft angiography. An adequate volume and rate of injection of contrast material are especially important, because many vein grafts are large and

difficult to fill. Significant errors in interpretation can result from underfilling of grafts. It is important to profile the proximal anastomosis and have adequate reflux into the aorta. It is easy to profile the graft origin when a ring marker is present by superimposing one side of the ring on the other (Fig. 4-36). This also makes identification of occlusion at the origin easier, because the stump is easier to see. It is a serious yet relatively common error to misinterpret a graft as being occluded at the proximal anastomosis when it has in fact not been adequately engaged. If there is any doubt, aortography should be performed. The body of the graft should be seen from at least two directions, and the distal anastomosis should be projected free of overlapping vessels.

Graft stenoses can occur at either anastomosis or in the body of the graft (Fig. 4-37). In the latter case, stenoses may be prone to occur at the site of venous valves (Fig. 4-38). The usual difficulty in determining the physiologic significance of coronary narrowing is compounded in saphenous grafts. One assumes that the size of a coronary artery is a function of the needed blood flow, but since there is no inherent correlation between the size of the vein and the needs of the myocardium supplied by it, one cannot make that same assumption about grafts (Fig. 4-39). For example, how significant is a 50% stenosis in a 4-mm vein that is connected to a 2-mm coronary artery? The answer will not be gleaned from the angiogram. High-grade stenoses are, of course, more likely to be physiologically significant, but the cineangiographer should always be wary of attaching significance to moderate graft stenoses.

Identification of narrowing at the distal anastomosis is often the most difficult part of the angiographic evaluation. In general, which view will best profile this region cannot be predicted prospectively, except that grafts to the LAD are almost always best visualized in the lateral view (Fig. 4-40A). Occasionally, a LAD graft is sutured in more from the side, in which case another view, usually a cranial left or cranial right anterior oblique view, is best (Fig. 4-40B, C). With grafts to other vessels, it may be difficult to see the distal anastomosis from two views (Fig. 4-41), and with grafts to the distal RCA it may be difficult to visualize the anastomosis at all. The suggested combinations listed in Table 4-1 should be liberally supplemented with other views depending on the individual anatomy.

The cineangiographer should be cautious of concluding that a graft is occluded proximally

Table 4-1 Recommended Views for Graft Distal Anastomoses

RCA and PDA	Cranial LAO, lateral
LAD	Lateral, cranial LAO, cranial RAO
Diagonal	Cranial LAO, cranial RAO
Obtuse marginal	RAO, lateral

LAD left anterior descending; LAO, left anterior oblique; PDA, posterior descending artery; RAO, right anterior descending; RCA, right coronary artery.

simply because contrast refluxes freely into it from the native coronary injection. Good forward flow through the native vessel can cause the same effect (Fig. 4-42). Graft occlusion must be proved by injection of the stump or aortography.

Sequential saphenous grafts to multiple vessels provide another challenge to the angiographer. These can involve combinations of two, three, or four native vessels. Stenosis or occlusion can occur in any limb or at any anastomosis, leaving the other limbs and anastomoses patent (Fig. 4-43). If there is antegrade flow into the grafted artery, the patent limbs may allow visualization of occluded native vessels even if part of the graft is occluded (Fig. 4-44).

Internal Mammary Grafts

Angiographic study of the LIMA is usually most easily accomplished with a left internal mammary catheter. Cannulation of the LIMA presents two challenges to the angiographer: engagement of the left subclavian artery and engagement of the LIMA itself. Unfortunately, the curve that makes it easiest to engage the subclavian is not always the curve that allows easy engagement of the LIMA. If difficulty is encountered either in engaging the subclavian or in advancing the LIMA catheter to the region of the LIMA, a right Judkins catheter can be used to enter the subclavian and advance a

(text continues on p. 101)

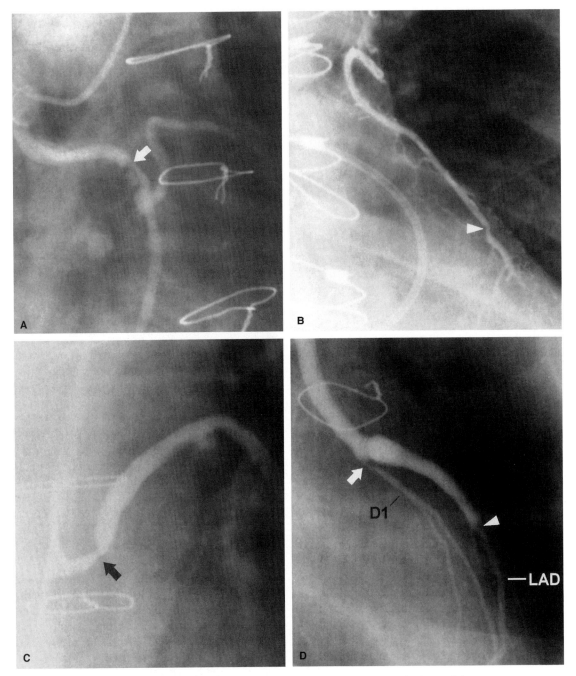

Figure 4-37. Graft stenoses. **(A)** Ulcerated stenosis in saphenous graft *(arrow)* just proximal to distal anastomosis. **(B)** Stenosis at distal anastomosis *(arrowhead)* of the left internal mammary artery to the left anterior descending. **(C)** Proximal saphenous vein graft stenosis *(arrow)*. **(D)** Sequential saphenous graft to the first diagonal (D1) and the left anterior descending (LAD). There is narrowing in D1 at the anastomosis *(arrow)* and in the segment of the graft between D1 and the LAD *(arrowhead)*.

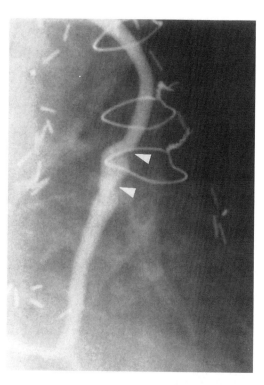

Figure 4-38. Focal dilatation at the site of a venous valve in a saphenous vein coronary graft. Residual valve material is probably present *(arrowheads).*

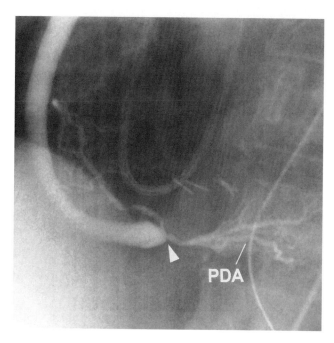

Figure 4-39. Saphenous vein graft to distal right coronary artery (RCA). Although there appears to be significant narrowing at the distal anastomosis *(arrowhead)*, the distal RCA is a very small vessel relative to the graft. (PDA, posterior descending artery.)

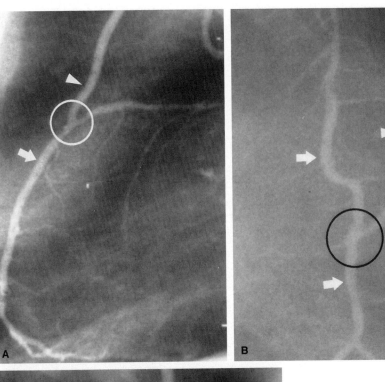

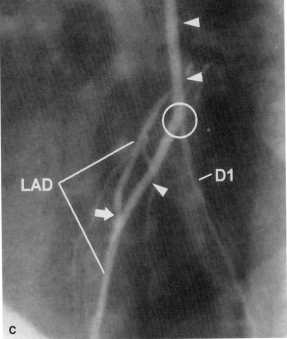

Figure 4-40. Graft from left internal mammary artery (LIMA) to left anterior descending (LAD). **(A)** Lateral view. The distal anastomosis *(circle)* is very well seen with the LIMA *(arrowhead)* projected clear of the LAD *(arrow)*. **(B)** In this patient, the distal anastomosis *(circle)* is seen better in the cranial left anterior oblique view because the LIMA *(arrowhead)* was sutured more into the side of the LAD *(arrows)*. **(C)** Sequential LIMA graft *(arrowheads)* to the first diagonal (D1) and the LAD. The anastomosis to the LAD is seen well *(arrow)*, but that to D1 is obscured by overlying LIMA *(circle)*.

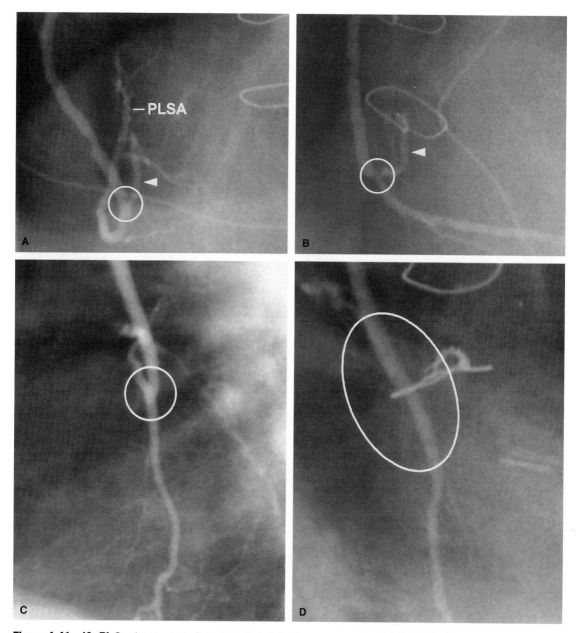

Figure 4-41. (A, B) Saphenous graft to the distal right coronary artery (RCA). The distal anastomosis *(circle)* is obscured in the right anterior oblique (RAO) view **(A)**, but nicely seen in the cranial left anterior oblique (LAO) view **(B)**. There is retrograde filling of the distal RCA *(arrowhead)*. **(C, D)** Saphenous graft to the first diagonal. The LAO view **(C)** shows the distal anastomosis *(circle)* with little overlap, but in the RAO view **(D)** one cannot discern where within the oval the anastomosis lies. (PLSA, posterolateral segment artery.)

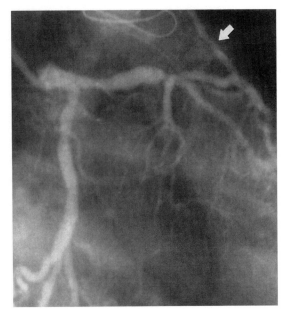

Figure 4-42. Injection of the left coronary shows reflux into a stenosis-free left internal mammary graft *(arrow)*. The maximum severity of stenosis in the proximal left anterior descending was about 50%.

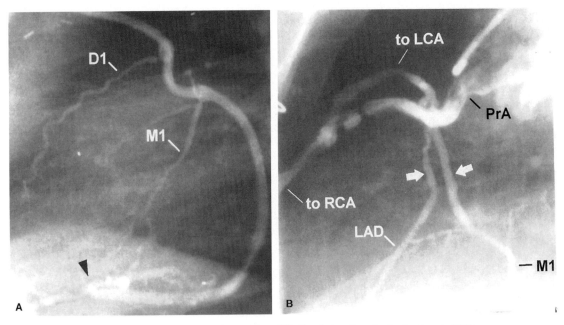

Figure 4-43. Sequential saphenous vein grafts. **(A)** Graft to the first diagonal (D1) continues to the first obtuse marginal (M1) and terminates on a posterolateral branch or the posterior descending *(arrowhead)*. **(B)** Complex sequential saphenous graft to both the right coronary artery (RCA) and left coronary artery (LCA). The proximal portion of the graft bifurcates into branches to the RCA and LCA. The LCA limb then splits into two branches *(arrows)*, one to the left anterior descending (LAD) and the other to the first obtuse marginal (M1). (PrA, proximal anastomosis.)

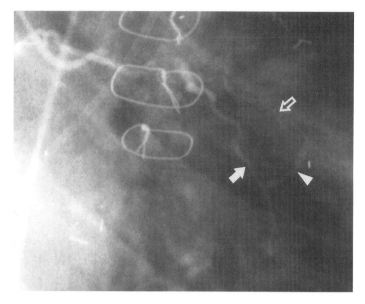

Figure 4-44. Sequential saphenous graft to a diagonal *(open arrow)* and a marginal *(solid arrow)*. The graft is occluded proximal to the diagonal. The segment of the graft between the two vessels remains patent *(arrowhead)*, allowing retrograde filling of the diagonal from the marginal.

guidewire into the axillary artery. In my experience, a standard 3-mm J-wire accomplishes this better than moveable-core J-wire. If this proves unsuccessful, a softer wire such as the Wholey wire or Terumo wire can be used. These must be advanced fairly far into the axillary artery to provide support to the catheter. The Judkins

catheter can then be exchanged for a LIMA catheter, which should slowly be withdrawn while applying counter-clockwise torque to engage the anteriorly arising LIMA (Fig. 4-45). Clockwise rotation frequently engages the thyrocervical trunk, causing neck pain when contrast material is injected. The cineangiographer

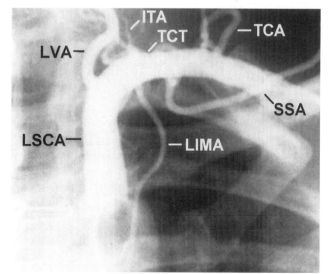

Figure 4-45. Left subclavian artery (LSCA) and its branches. The left vertebral artery (LVA), left internal mammary artery (LIMA), and thyrocervical trunk (TCT) arise directly from the LSCA. The inferior thyroid artery (ITA), transcervical artery (TCA), and suprascapular artery (SSA) come from the TCT. Posterior orientation of the tip on the internal mammary catheter will result in cannulation of the TCT.

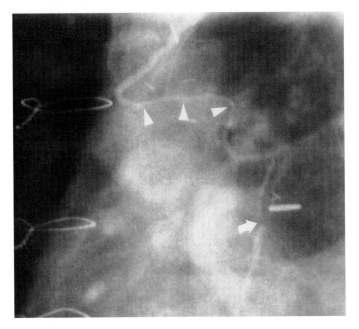

Figure 4-46. Left internal mammary artery (LIMA) graft to the left anterior descending. In addition to a stenosis at the distal anastomosis *(arrow)*, there is severe diffuse narrowing of a substantial portion of the LIMA *(arrowheads)*. At reoperation, these conditions were found to be caused by involvement of the LIMA by pericardial inflammation.

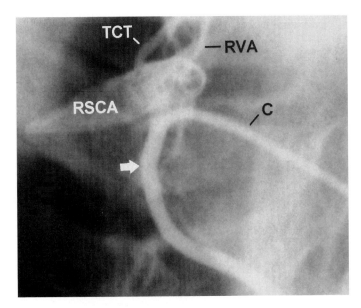

Figure 4-47. Selective injection of the right internal mammary artery *(arrow)* with reflux into the right subclavian artery (RSCA). (C, catheter; RVA, right vertebral artery; TCT, thyrocervical trunk.)

must also be extremely careful not to poke the wire or catheter into the left vertebral artery, or untoward circumstances may result. The word of the day here is "gentle."

After the body of the LIMA has been seen in one or perhaps two views, angiographic evaluation should focus on the distal anastomosis. It is better not to try to see the entire LIMA on every shot, because this requires a significant amount of panning and makes it difficult to maintain a uniform x-ray field. The result can be underexposure of the distal portion of the graft and the distal anastomosis because of the presence of a substantial amount of lung in the field. It is critical to visualize the region of the distal anastomosis and adjacent coronary artery, because this is where the majority of problems occur (Fig. 4-46; see Fig. 4-40*A*) Stenoses in the body of the LIMA are unusual and may be related to technical problems with the clipping of side branches or involvement of the vessel by pericardial inflammation (see Fig. 4-46).

RIMA grafts are less frequently encountered than LIMA grafts (Fig. 4-47). If the RIMA is used as a free graft, cannulation is accomplished in the same manner as with saphenous grafts. In situ RIMA grafts usually go to either the RCA or the LAD. They can be cannulated in much the same way as the LIMA by using a right Judkins catheter to engage the innominate artery, passing a guidewire into the right subclavian artery, and exchanging it for a LIMA catheter. Care should be taken to minimize trauma to the right common carotid artery caused by inadvertently passing the wire or catheter into it.

EVALUATION OF THE CORONARY ARTERIES AFTER INTERVENTION

Coronary intervention tends to cause rather severe perturbations in the wall of the affected

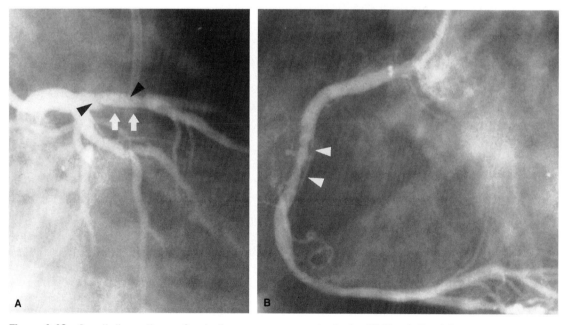

Figure 4-48. Small dissections after balloon coronary angioplasty. **(A)** Two intimal flaps *(arrowheads)* and a linear extraluminal collection of contrast material *(arrows)* are present after angioplasty of the proximal left anterior descending. **(B)** There is a long, parallel dissection *(arrowheads)* of the mid right coronary artery without apparent significant luminal compromise.

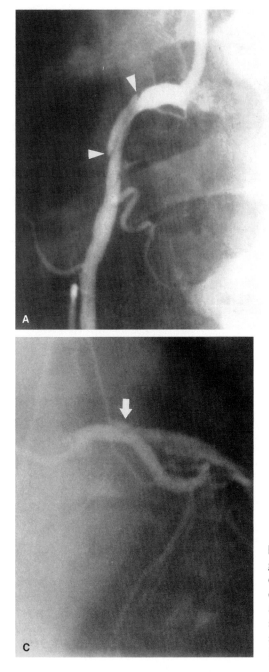

Figure 4-49. Significant dissections after balloon angioplasty. **(A)** Long dissection of the proximal right coronary artery *(between arrowheads)* with significant luminal narrowing. Angiograms made **(B)** before and **(C)** after angioplasty of an apparently mild stenosis of the proximal left anterior descending show significant dissection of the distal left main *(arrow).*

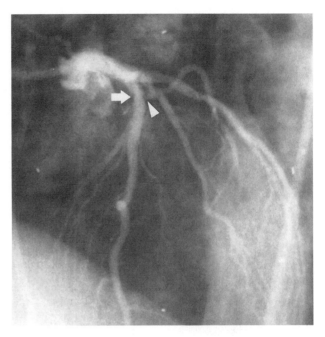

Figure 4-50. Side branch occlusion after angioplasty of the left anterior descending (LAD). Although there is minimal residual narrowing in the LAD *(arrow)*, the second diagonal, which was not narrowed before the procedure, is almost occluded at its origin *(arrowhead)*.

vessel, frequently resulting in a less than straight-forward angiographic appearance. Evaluation of intervention sites should include assessment of both the severity of residual narrowing and the presence or absence of any complication such as dissection, clot formation, or distal embolization.

Coronary narrowing is even more difficult to evaluate after *balloon angioplasty* than it is before. This is no surprise considering that balloon angioplasty works in part by plaque fracture, leaving a poorly defined lumen that can result in a hazy appearance. Small linear dissections are commonly seen and are usually of no immediate clinical consequence (Fig. 4-48). More important are the so-called spiral dissections (Fig. 4-49). These can involve large segments of the vessel at, proximal to, or distal to the dilatation site and may be associated with diminished flow distal to the lesion and acute occlusion of the dilated vessel or its branches. Side vessels can become temporarily or permanently occluded during the procedure or be left with significant stenosis even if they were normal before the procedure (Fig. 4-50).[15]

Coronary atherectomy tends to result in a cleaner-appearing image and better definition of the vessel wall than does balloon angioplasty (Fig. 4-51). Significant dissections do occur, however, especially if too large a device is used. Damage to the vessel distal to the atherectomy site can occur from the nose cone of the device, and can cause stenosis late after the procedure that clinically mimics restenosis (Fig. 4-52).

Laser angioplasty usually results in a small lumen because the laser probes are fairly small. Most of these patients undergo further balloon dilatation, which dictates the angiographic appearance. As with any other intervention, dissection and occlusion can occur.

Thrombus is occasionally seen after any type of intervention and appears as one or more filling defects in the lumen, either proximal, at, or distal to the stenosis (Fig. 4-53). If they are small, thrombi may be difficult to differentiate angiographically from small dissections. For a more detailed description of the postintervention appearance of the coronary arteries, the reader is referred to Popma's text.[16]

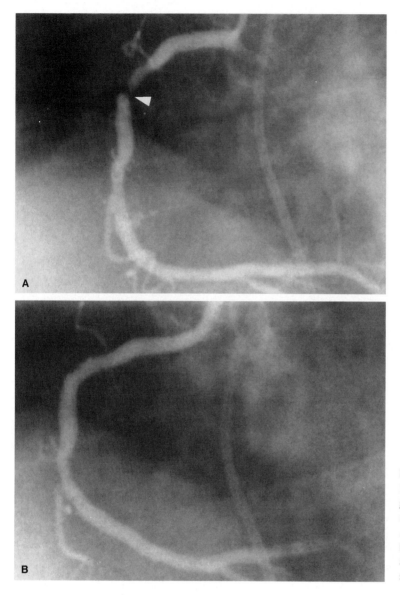

Figure 4-51. Directional coronary atherectomy. **(A)** High-grade stenosis in the proximal right coronary artery *(arrowhead)*. **(B)** There is minimal narrowing after atherectomy, and the lumen appears fairly smooth.

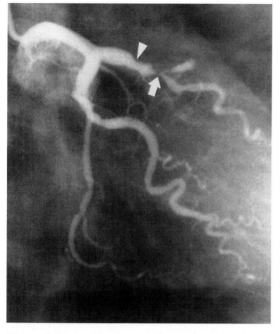

Figure 4-52. Nose cone damage from directional atherectomy. Moderate narrowing is present at the previous atherectomy site in the proximal left anterior descending (LAD; *arrowhead*). Distally, there is severe narrowing of the LAD involving the origin of the first diagonal *(arrow)*. This area was not stenotic before atherectomy.

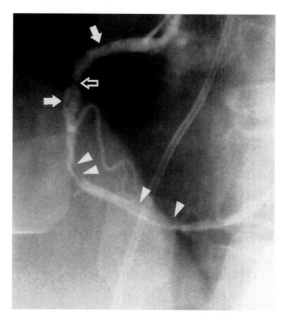

Figure 4-53. Extensive dissection of the right coronary artery after balloon angioplasty. Thin linear filling defects *(solid arrows)* are seen proximal and distal to the dilatation site *(open arrow)* and are most consistent with intimal flaps. Distally, there are larger filling defects *(arrowheads)*, more suggestive of thrombus.

References

1. Arnett EN, Isner JM, Redwood DR, et al. Coronary artery narrowing in coronary heart disease: comparison of cineangiographic and necropsy findings. Ann Intern Med 1979;91:350.

2. Levin DC, Gardiner GA. Complex and simple coronary artery stenoses: a new way to interpret coronary angiograms based on morphologic features of lesions. Radiology 1987;164:675.

3. Higano ST, Nishimura RA. Intravascular ultrasonography. Curr Probl Cardiol 1994; 19:28.

4. Zack PM, Ischinger T, Aker UT, et al. The occurrence of angiographically detected intracoronary thrombus in patients with unstable angina pectoris. Am Heart J 1984; 108:1408.

5. Rentrop P, Blanke H, Karsch KR, et al. Selective intracoronary thrombolysis in acute myocardial infarction and unstable angina pectoris. Circulation 1981;63:307.

6. Morphogenesis of occluding coronary artery thrombosis. Arch Pathol 1965;80:256.

7. Markis JE, Joffe CD, Cohn PF, et al. Clinical significance of coronary arterial ectasia. Am J Cardiol 1976;37:217.

8. Melish ME, Hicks RM, Dean AC, Marchette NJ. Endemic and epidemic Kawasaki syndrome. Pediatr Res 1981;15:617.

9. Heggveit HA. Syphilitic aortitis: a clinicopathologic autopsy study of 100 cases, 1950 to 1960. Circulation 1964;29:346.

10. Yasue H, Akinori T, Nagao M, et al. Pathogenesis of angina pectoris in patients with one-vessel disease: possible role of dynamic coronary obstruction. Am Heart J 1986; 112:263.

11. Kuhn FE, Mohler ER, Satler LF, et al.

High-density lipoprotein influences acetylcholine induced coronary vasoreactivity. Am J Cardiol 1991;68:1425.

12. Kramer JR, Kitazume H, Proudfit WL, Sones FM: Clinical significance of isolated coronary bridges: benign and frequent condition involving the left anterior descending artery. Am Heart J 1982;103:283.

13. Green CE, Kelley JM, Higgins CB, et al. Acquired coronary to bronchial communication: a possible cause of coronary steal. Cathet Cardiovasc Diagn 1980;7:191.

14. Loop FD, Lytle W, Cosgrove DM, et al. Influence of the internal mammary graft on 10-year survival and other cardiac events. N Engl J Med 1986;314:1.

15. Ciampricotti R, El Gamal M, van Gelder B, et al. Coronary angioplasty of bifurcational lesions without protection of large side branches. Cathet Cardiovasc Diagn 1992;27:191.

16. Popma JJ, Leon MB, Topol EJ. Atlas of interventional cardiology. Philadelpha: WB Saunders, 1994.

Coronary Cinematography, by Curtis E. Green.
Lippincott–Raven Publishers, © 1995.

CHAPTER *FIVE*

Estimation of Coronary Artery Narrowing

The coronary arteries are among the most difficult vessels to image, and the images are difficult to interpret, especially with regard to estimation of severity of narrowing. The traditional method for describing coronary stenoses has been in terms of relative luminal narrowing. More recent techniques have focused either on more precise measurement of luminal diameter or on calculation of cross-sectional area. All techniques for estimating coronary narrowing are affected by anatomic, radiographic, and physiologic factors. These factors can affect determination of both relative stenosis and absolute diameter.

The most commonly used method for estimating coronary narrowing is determination of percent diameter stenosis. Despite limitations, this remains the most popular technique because of the facility with which it can be done and because, in the clinical setting, the information it provides is usually adequate for decision making, especially if it is combined with the results of physiologic tests.

DETERMINATION OF RELATIVE STENOSIS

To measure percent diameter narrowing, the diameter of a stenotic segment of the coronary artery is compared with a reference segment, which is assumed to be of normal caliber. The ratio of the diameter of the vessel at the stenosis to the reference diameter is then expressed to whatever precision is appropriate for the particular stenosis. For a well-demarcated stenosis in the middle of an otherwise normal-caliber vessel, this may be to the nearest 10%. With less well-defined lesions or

109

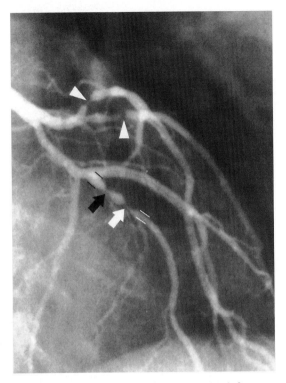

Figure 5-1. Measuring stenoses in the left anterior descending and first diagonal branch *(arrowheads)* and sequential stenoses in the inferior branch of the first obtuse marginal *(arrows)*. Choosing the reference diameter for the marginal lesions is more difficult because the vessel tapers significantly over a short distance. Percent stenosis will be higher if the *black lines* are chosen and lower if the *white lines* are used.

diffuse reference segment disease, ranges are more realistic (e.g., 20%–40%, 50%–75%, >90%) (Fig. 5-1). Cine film resolution limits preclude visualization of the lumen in any but very large vessels if diameter narrowing is greater than 85% to 90%, which makes the so-called 99% stenosis somewhat apocryphal. The tendency to refer to 95% and 99% narrowing is reminiscent of what the Danish comedian and pianist Victor Borge termed "inflationary language," in which every word containing a number was arbitrarily increased by one, so that "wonderful" became "twoderful" and "before" became "befive." This same technique seems to have been adopted by a substantial number of angiographers without giving credit to Mr. Borge.

Difficulties of Measurement

There are several problems with measurement of relative stenosis that should be immediately apparent. First and foremost is the selection of the reference segment. Unrecognized narrowing of the reference segment results in underestimation of the stenosis (Fig. 5-2). Because diffuse disease has been shown in pathologic studies to be very common,[1–3] underestimation is a frequent problem. Ectasia of the reference segment can result in overestimation of narrowing for the opposite reason (Fig. 5-3). Similarly, if the cineangiographer is forced to use as a reference segment an area of vessel that is located far distal to the stenosis or after a large branch, the validity of the reference segment is also suspect. Underfilling of the vessel distal to an obstruction also causes underestimation of percent diameter narrowing if the distal vessel is used as the reference segment. This can be seen, for instance, if there is streaming of contrast material along the dependent wall of the vessel distal to a high-grade stenosis or if there is collateral flow into the distal vessel with dilution of contrast material by unopacified blood from the collaterals.[4] Changes in vascular tone can result in inaccurate estimation of narrowing by causing superimposed spasm (Fig. 5-4) or preferential dilatation of the reference segment.

A second issue involves how a given lesion is measured. Unfortunately, many angiographers simply look at the lesion and visually compare it

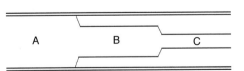

Figure 5-2. Effect of diffuse narrowing on estimation of severity of stenosis. If normal vessel luminal diameter is at region A, then narrowing in region B would be graded as 50% stenosis and that in region C as 75% stenosis. If the entire vessel is narrowed to the extent present in region B, however, region C will appear to be narrowed only 50%, and the severity of narrowing will be underestimated.

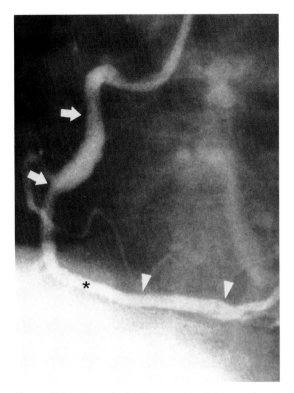

Figure 5-3. Ectasia in the proximal *(arrows)* and distal *(arrowheads)* portions of the right coronary make selection of a reference diameter difficult. The area of narrower but smooth vessel between *(asterisk)* may be normal in caliber.

with the reference segment. This results in inaccurate and poorly reproducible results and has no doubt led to the misinterpretation of many studies. For example, in the Coronary Artery Surgery Study, investigators found that, if one observer reported a stenosis of greater than 50% in the left main coronary artery, a second observer reported no stenosis 18.6% of the time.[5] Similarly, with lesions reported as 70% or greater by one observer, the second observer agreed in only 72.1% of segments. A study by DeRouen and colleagues[6] using 11 observers and 10 arterial segments showed a standard deviation of 18% for visualization of all segments, varying from 8% in the proximal right coronary artery to 28.5% in the diagonal arteries. Variation can be decreased by consensus opinion[7] and is less severe with lesions of less than 20% or more than 80% stenosis.[8] Visual overestimation of stenoses

is of particular importance with regard to the decision to pursue coronary intervention. According to a prominent interventional cardiologist, there is a strong temptation to add 20 percentage points to the predilatation assessment and take off 20 points after dilatation.

The eye, however, is not such a bad judge of the vessel edge, and if some mechanism to transfer the size of the stenosis lumen to the reference segment is used, a reasonable degree of precision and reproducibility can be obtained. Although this can be accomplished with electronic digital calipers, hand-held electrocardiographic calipers work well for day-to-day use. Considering the inherent limitations of angiographic technique, particularly the difficulty in determining normal reference diameter, it may be true that clinically, there is no significantly greater accuracy with sophisticated techniques than with calipers. This is especially relevant if the philosophy that ranges of narrowing should be used is adopted. Given these limitations, is there really any difference between a 70% (or even a 60%) stenosis as determined with electrocardiographic calipers and a 73% stenosis as read on the digital calipers? To a large degree, in clinical work the precise amount of stenosis is irrelevant so long as the narrowing is greater than that usually associated with clinical significance. Furthermore, making clinical decisions based solely on the angiographic appearance of a lesion is hazardous.

The third major difficulty in measuring percent diameter narrowing arises from the fact that coronary stenoses are rarely symmetrical in shape. In a study of 200 sections of atheromatous coronary artery, Vlodaver and Edward[9] found a central lumen in only 30.5% , whereas 40.5% has an eccentric polymorphous lumen and 29% had an eccentric slit-like lumen. This is an issue regardless of whether the worst view or the average of two views is used (Fig. 5-5). Calculation of percent area narrowing adds another element of uncertainty because it requires a geometric model (e.g., circle, ellipse, rectangle), which is probably inaccurate. Computer-assisted techniques for measuring relative stenosis have resulted in a higher degree of consistency but are still affected by these basic limitations.

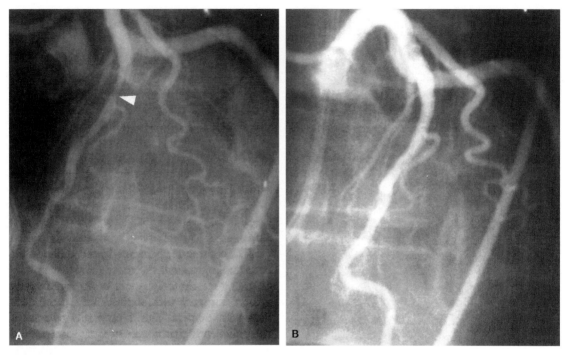

Figure 5-4. Spontaneous spasm mimicking a stenosis. Views of the left coronary artery were made **(A)** before and **(B)** after nitroglycerin administration with spasm just proximal to the second diagonal artery *(arrowhead)*.

Physiologic Considerations

In addition to the problems with the actual measuring of stenoses, there are limitations that derive from physiologic factors, so that even if accurate measurements are available, there may be a poor correlation with physiologic parameters.[10]

There are many reasons why relative stenosis alone may not adequately predict the significance of a coronary lesion. For example, although a stenosis of 50% is required to reduce coronary flow reserve with normal coronary blood flow, flow reserve can be decreased by a 30% to 40% stenosis when blood flow is maximized.[11] Similar results have been obtained in dogs: Higgins and coworkers, looking at absolute coronary blood flow, found that under normal flow conditions, a stenosis of 80% was required to reduce flow, but under conditions of maximal vasodilatation, only a 43% stenosis was required.[12]

Morphology of the stenosis plays a consider-able role as well. Cross-sectional area is the most important factor in determining resistance to flow.[13] Length alone has a significantly smaller effect,[13–15] but multiple stenoses close together have a greater effect than a single stenosis of equivalent length because of energy loss at the entrance and exit points of the stenoses.[16,17] Other factors include lesion asymmetry[18,19] and

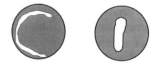

Figure 5-5. Effect of stenosis morphology on estimation of narrowing. The asymmetric stenosis depicted on the right measures 84% in its narrow-est dimension and 38% at its widest. Despite obvious significant luminal compromise, the stenosis on the left, because of its shape, mea-sures no more than 31% in any dimension.

the shape of the entrance and exit portions of the stenosis.[20]

Epicardial blood flow is also affected by physiologic factors such as vasomotor tone,[21] perfusion pressure (systemic diastolic blood pressure), and coronary bed resistance.

QUANTITATIVE CORONARY ANGIOGRAPHY

The need for more objective measurement of stenoses for coronary intervention and atherosclerosis regression studies has led to the development of computer-assisted techniques. These have been used to provide more consistency and objectivity in the calculation of relative narrowing, but more importantly, they also provide a means for determining absolute stenosis diameter and, in some cases, minimal cross-sectional area. Quantitative coronary angiography (QCA) also provides, in many cases, better characterization of the state of disease. It is not widely used for clinical work for several reasons, including long processing time and the cost of the equipment required. Also, some stenoses cannot be quantified because of factors such as poor x-ray technique, overlapping vessels, or side branches. Furthermore, as discussed previously, the exact degree of narrowing is not the only factor determining the importance of a stenosis. Despite these problems, QCA has become an important tool for the investigator, and, in some cases, it can play an important clinical role, especially if the objectivity of the angiographer is suspect or there is disagreement about the severity of a stenosis.

Technique

Computer-assisted analysis of coronary angiograms requires excellent image quality: computers cannot make inadequate images into accurate information. As data analysts like to say, "garbage in, garbage out." Most analysis is done off-line for convenience and time considerations and thus uses cine film. On-line techniques are available in catheterization laboratories equipped with digital systems to aid in immediate clinical decisions, but in the author's experience these are infrequently used for anything more than a sophisticated video replay system.

The first step is digitization of the image, either simultaneous with film acquisition or off-line. Post facto digitization requires an excellent-quality projector and digitizing camera if information is not to be lost. After the information is in digital form, the computer can process the image, allowing edge enhancement, changes in contrast, and measurements. Depending on the particular system, a variable amount of operator interaction is required, but at the very least the operator must choose the area of interest and designate which part of the vessel represents the lesion, which part the reference segment, and what to use as a calibration standard (Fig. 5-6). It must be kept in mind, however, that these numbers can be no better than the image from which they were derived. In fact, it has been estimated that the variation in quantitative measurements that results from angiographic quality is two to four times greater than that resulting from the analysis itself.[22]

The factors affecting *image quality* were discussed in detail in Chapter 1. From a practical standpoint, the most important are the beam energy (kVp) and the concentration of iodine in the vessel. High kVp causes increased quantum mottle and poor radiographic contrast, both of which decrease sharpness of the vessel edge. Low iodine concentration also produces poor vessel contrast and can result from a number of operator-controlled factors, including use of contrast material with a low iodine content, inadequate injection rate and volume, and mixing of blood and iodine in the syringe. Anatomic factors such as poor flow across a severe stenosis and collateral filling of the distal vessel can also adversely affect image quality. Vessels and catheters near the edge of the image intensifier may be distorted by pincushion effect, and any vessel that is not perpendicular to the x-ray beam is distorted to some degree (Fig. 5-7).

Image (frame) selection is completely operator-dependent and has a major effect on QCA. Ideally, a frame at end-diastole, with the vessel completely filled and free of any superimposition of another vessel, should be used. If there is

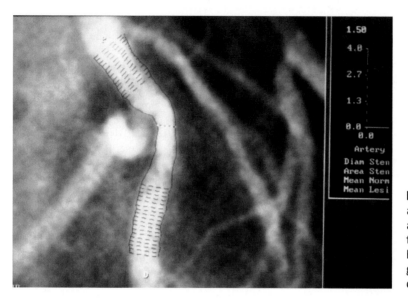

Figure 5-6. Computer-generated quantitative analysis of a discrete stenosis in an obtuse marginal. The computer has tracked the vessel margins and chosen a minimal diameter.

overlap, it may be necessary to use a frame at other than end-diastole; however, frames that are taken near end-systole may cause vessel size to be badly underestimated.

Changes in *vasomotor tone* can affect measurement of the lesions and the reference seg-ments. This can induce a large error, especially if lesions are being compared between studies, as in a study of coronary regression or of restenosis after intervention. Because of this problem, long-term studies require the use of a vasodilator to ensure maximal vessel dilatation.

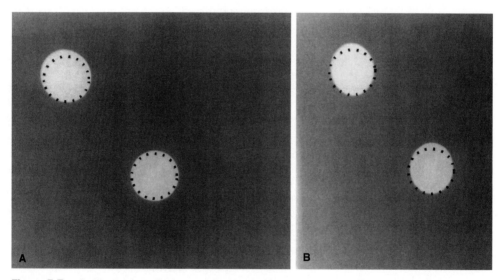

Figure 5-7. Radiographs of two coins demonstrate distortion. **(A)** Straight posteroanterior view. Overlying dashed circles show that the image of the coin at the outer edge of the intensifier has an oval shape because of the pincushion effect. The coin in the center is almost round. **(B)** A 30-degree left anterior oblique view results in distortion of both coins, because they are no longer perpendicular to the x-ray beam.

Measurement of absolute vessel dimensions requires a *calibration standard* unless the study is performed biplane, in which case radiographic magnification can be calculated if the proper parameters are recorded (mainly tube angles and source-to-image distances). Because of its proximity to the coronary arteries, the angiographic catheter is the most convenient calibration standard, but its use has several limitations. First, the catheter is not usually in exactly the same plane as the coronary artery and therefore may be magnified differently. This difference in magnification changes according to the specific view and the specific vessels. For example, in the right anterior oblique view, there should be little difference in magnification between the catheter and the LAD, but the left circumflex is more magnified than the catheter because it is closer to the x-ray tube. Catheter composition is also important. For QCA, it has been found that catheters composed of woven Dacron have the least variation between calculated and actual size. Polyvinylchloride and polyurethane catheters are less good, but acceptable; nylon catheters are unsatisfactory.[22] Variation in actual size can be found among supposedly identical catheters from the same manufacturer. Measured size is also affected by the presence of contrast material in the catheter. It is recommended that, for a catheter to be acceptable for QCA, the standard deviation of a series of measurements made at various contrast concentrations and beam energies should be less than 0.03 mm (0.1 Fr).[22] There is frequently also a disparity in apparent size between different parts of the catheter; this seems to be a result of region-to-region variations in film density. This raises the obvious question as to which part of the picture shows the true catheter size. The usual policy is to opt for the widest-appearing part; however, no matter which part is used, the most important thing is to be consistent and to use the same technique for all studies.

With the possible exception of image quality, the most important factor affecting quantitative measurements, relative and absolute, is the limitation of angiographic imaging that results from the nature of the atherosclerotic process. The fact is that no matter how good an image and how sophisticated the computer, there is no way of absolutely knowing that an apparently normal segment is not actually narrowed or dilated. This affects relative measurements more than absolute measurements because selection of the reference segment is critical with the former, just as it is with manual determination of relative narrowing. Similar difficulty arises when determining lesion length. It should also be remembered that these techniques are computer assisted, and frequent user input is required when the computer does not track the vessel perimeter properly. The more the cineangiographer relies on manual correction of vessel edges, the more potential there is for interjection of bias.

SUMMARY

For the day-to-day interpretation of coronary angiograms, manual determination of relative stenosis is adequate, providing some type of caliper is used and some semblance of objectivity is maintained, and providing the angiographic results are correlated with symptoms and with the results of physiologic tests. Scientific studies demand a more rigorous approach, which, for the most part, can be provided by QCA. Regardless of the degree of sophistication, computer-assisted techniques are still subject to the inherent limitations of angiography, and no QCA system can accurately analyze a poor-quality image.

REFERENCES

1. Arnett EN, Isner JM, Redwood DR, et al. Coronary artery narrowing in coronary heart disease: comparison of cineangiographic and necropsy findings. Ann Intern Med 1979;91:350.
2. Roberts WC, Buja LM. The frequency and significance of coronary arterial thrombi and other observations in fatal acute myocardial infarction. A study of 107 necropsy patients. Am J Med 1972;52:425.
3. Isner JM, Wu M, Virmani R, et al. Comparison of degrees of coronary arterial luminal narrowing determined by visual inspection of histologic sections under magnification among three independent observers and

comparison to that obtained by video planimetry. An analysis of 559 five-millimeter segments of 61 coronary arteries from eleven patients. Lab Invest 1980; 5:566.

4. Levin DC, Baltaxe HA, Sos TA. Potential sources of error in coronary arteriography. II: In interpretation of the study. AJR Am J Roentgenol 1975;124:386.

5. Fisher LD, Judkins MP, Lespèrance J, et al. Reproducibility of coronary arteriographic reading in the Coronary Artery Surgery Study (CASS). Cathet Cardiovasc Diagn 1982;8:565.

6. DeRouen TA, Murray JA, Owen W. Variability in the analysis of coronary arteriograms. Circulation 1977;55:324.

7. Zir LM. Observer variability in coronary angiography (editorial note). Int J Cardiol 1983;3:171.

8. Shub C, Vlietstra RE, Smith HC, et al. The unpredictable progression of symptomatic coronary artery disease. A serial clinical-angiographic analysis. Mayo Clin Proc 1981;56:155.

9. Vlodaver Z, Edward JE. Pathology of coronary atherosclerosis. Prog Cardiovasc Dis 1971;14:256.

10. White CW, Wright CB, Doty DB, et al. Does visual interpretation of the coronary arteriogram predict the physiologic importance of a coronary stenosis? N Engl J Med 1984;310:819.

11. Dietze W, Mittmann U, Schmier J, Wirth RH. Effects of coronary stenosis and mean aortic pressure on coronary blood flow, poststenotic coronary pressure, and reactive hyperemia. Basic Res Cardiol 1976;71:309.

12. Higgins CB, Kelley MJ, Green CE, et al. Physiologic-angiographic correlates of coronary arterial stenosis in resting and intensely vasodilated states. Invest Radiol 1982;17:444.

13. Lipscomb K, Hooten S. Effect of stenotic dimensions and blood flow on the hemodynamic significance of model coronary arterial stenoses. Am J Cardiol 1978;42:781.

14. Logan SE. On the fluid mechanics of human coronary artery stenosis. IEEE Trans Biomed Eng 1975;22:327.

15. Fiddian RV, Byar D, Edwards EA. Factors affecting flow through a stenosed vessel. Arch Surg 1964;88:83.

16. Sabbah HN, Stein PD. Hemodynamics of multiple versus single 50 percent coronary arterial stenoses. Am J Cardiol 1982;50:276.

17. Feldman RL, Nichols WW, Pepine CJ, et al. The coronary hemodynamics of left main and branch coronary stenoses. The effects of reduction in stenosis diameter, stenosis length, and number of stenoses. J Thorac Cardiovasc Surg 1979;77:377.

18. Young DF, Tsai FY. Flow characteristics in models of arterial stenoses. I: Steady flow. J Biomech 1973;6:395.

19. Young DF, Tsai FY. Flow characteristics in models of arterial stenoses. II: Unsteady flow. J Biomech 1973;6:547.

20. Clark C. The propagation of turbulence produced by a stenosis. J Biomech 1980; 13:591.

21. Feldman RL, Pepine CJ. Determination of residual regional flow during acute coronary occlusion in conscious man (abstract). J Am Coll Cardiol 1983;1:684.

22. Reiber JHC, Serruys PW, Slager CJ. Quantitative coronary and left ventricular cineangiography. Dordrecht, Netherlands: Martinus Nijhoff, 1986:129.

Coronary Cinematography, by Curtis E. Green.
Lippincott–Raven Publishers, © 1995.

CHAPTER SIX

Optimizing Image Quality

All of the discussion so far about x-ray and angiographic techniques has focused on each area individually. This chapter attempts to tie all of these factors together and provide a framework for producing consistently good cineangiograms.

TECHNICAL FACTORS

The Ideal Exposure

Certain radiographic parameters contribute to image quality. These are described in detail in Chapter 1 but can be summarized by describing the features of a theoretical ideal exposure:

- low beam energy (kVp) to increase image contrast
- short exposure time to minimize motion artifact
- high tube current to decrease noise
- small focal spot to decrease geometric unsharpness.

Unfortunately, these goals may be mutually exclusive to some degree, and there are no absolute rules for determining which are more important in a given circumstance. As a result, much of the art of coronary angiography consists of knowing when and what to trade among factors. The following discussion attempts to clarify and put into perspective the issues faced when trying to optimize image quality.

117

Image Intensifier Mode

In the technical data published by x-ray equipment manufacturers are tables showing the spatial resolution capabilities of the image intensifiers. The spatial resolutions shown vary from about 2 line pairs per millimeter on low magnification mode to more than 5 line pairs per millimeter on high magnification mode, theoretically allowing resolution of objects smaller than 0.2 mm. The increase in spatial resolution with decreasing field size (higher magnification) suggests that the highest possible magnification should be used for maximum spatial resolution. The problem with this conclusion is that the advertised numbers were obtained under ideal circumstances: a resolution grid placed directly against the image intensifier, low kVp, and no motion. This is quite different from the clinical situation, in which the intensifier is displaced from the heart, the kVp is undoubtedly higher, and the coronaries are moving. It is unreasonable to expect to see the same spatial resolution with a patient as with a line pair phantom. To further complicate matters, the trade-off in technical factors is different for each patient and even for each different view. For example, with an 80-pound patient, high-quality images in high magnification mode could reasonably be expected, even in the caudal left anterior oblique view; with a 300-pound patient, resolution may be considerably less in high magnification mode than in even the lowest magnification mode on every view. The major reason for this paradox is, of course, that the higher-magnification view requires a higher kVp, which results in diminished contrast resolution (Fig. 6-1). Remember, bigger is not always sharper.

Beam Geometry

There are two beneficial results of keeping the image intensifier close to the patient's chest. Penumbra (edge gradient or geometric unsharpness) is increased as the object-to-image distance is increased (see Fig. 1-15). In addition, the x-ray dose required to maintain proper film exposure increases proportional to the square of the distance between the x-ray source and the image, so that if the source-to-image distance is doubled, the radiation dose must be quadrupled. Maintaining the shortest possible object-to-image distance by keeping the intensifier close to the chest wall reduces both penumbra and x-ray tube output requirements.

Frame Rate

It seems to be an accepted practice to use 30 frames per second for adult cineangiography; however, some angiographers still prefer 60 frames per second because there is less flicker and the image appears smoother. There are two obvious disadvantages to this practice. First, because twice as many exposures are made, the x-ray tube output must be increased, causing greater exposure to both patient and operator. Second, x-ray tube heating is greater, and there is less time for cooling. This can result in a higher kVp technique, with resulting poorer contrast, greater noise, and overall image degradation: a high price for smoothness. In general, use of 60 frames per second should be restricted to angiography of pediatric patients, coronary angiography in small adults with fast heart rates, and pulmonary angiography.

Pulse Width

To photograph moving objects, it is best to use the shortest possible exposure time to decrease motion artifact. For the photographer, the main limits on exposure time are the amount of light available and the aperture of the camera. As the exposure time is shortened, the aperture must be opened in a reciprocal fashion or the film will be underexposed. Of course, larger apertures result in less depth of field, so there are compromises to be made.

With cineangiography, depth of field is not important because the image is flat; therefore, the aperture is usually wide open ($\approx$f/2) and fixed. The amount of light available to work with, however, is limited, because x-ray generators do not have unlimited capacity and image

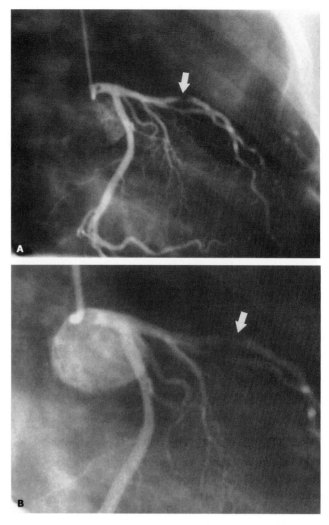

Figure 6-1. Paradoxical decrease in resolution in high magnification mode. Right anterior oblique views of the left coronary artery in (**A**) medium magnification mode and (**B**) high magnification mode. Primarily because of higher peak kilovoltage, the edges of the stenosis in the mid left anterior descending *(arrow)* are seen more clearly at lower magification.

intensifiers are not 100% efficient. With the fixed aperture of most systems, the only way to compensate for a short exposure time (pulse width) is to increase either tube current (mA) or kVp. As discussed previously, it is much more efficient to increase exposure by raising kVp because less heat is generated than when mA is increased. Given a fixed pulse width, most generators increase mA first and then raise kVp, but the extent to which they can do this is limited. Therefore, when pulse width becomes very short, tube heating becomes a significant issue and image quality is bound to suffer. There is one x-ray system in which the aperture is auto-

matically changed electronically; if the kVp goes above or below preset values, the aperture opens or closes, respectively. The drawback to this system is that when the aperture opens, the dose decreases and the image may become noisier. Whether it is better to have more noise because of lower dose than because of higher kVp is unclear.

From a practical standpoint, pulse widths between 4 and 8 msec are usually satisfactory for coronary angiography. If longer than 8 msec is required to maintain proper film exposure, the cineangiographer should consider increasing focal spot size or decreasing image intensifier magnification. Pulse widths shorter than 4 msec result in little decrease in motion unsharpness at a relatively high cost in tube loading.

Focal Spot

Ideally, a small focal spot should be used to decrease penumbra. This is especially important if there is geometric magnification resulting from displacement of the image intensifier away from the chest wall. Unfortunately, the low heat capacity and kilowatt loading of the small focal spot place severe constraints on this goal, especially when trying to keep exposure time down. For example, with a Philips SRM x-ray tube, the small focal spot (0.6 mm) is rated for 35 kW, and the large focal spot (1.2 mm) is rated for 100 kW. This means that less mA can be generated with the small focal spot, so that increases in exposure require adjustments in pulse width or kVp. The first adds motion unsharpness, and the latter decreases image contrast. A compromise approach is to use small focal spot until the kVp exceeds 90 at a pulse width of 8 msec. At that point, it is probably better to increase focal spot size rather than go to a longer pulse width. These numbers are not hard and fast, however, and may vary from system to system and with the personal preference of the angiographer.

Cine Run Time

As described previously, this term refers to the maximum length of time that the cine camera is allowed to run. Because the generator calculates its potential heat load and thus the best x-ray technique based in part on this number, it has a significant influence on whether or not maximum potential is achieved. In simplistic terms, if the cine run is set for 20 seconds, the generator will set the mA lower and the kVp higher than if the maximum time were to be 10 seconds, because the latter run potentially generates only one half as much heat. This is independent of how long the subsequent run actually is; the generator assumes that it will go a full 20 seconds. Because of this situation, it makes sense to limit maximum run time to no more than 8 to

10 seconds for coronary work. Even at this time limit, many systems allow for some overrun; it is very rare that a run is cut off prematurely. This is almost a penalty-free modification, but it must be done by the x-ray repair technician and is not changeable at the console.

Angiographic Technique

Although the technical factors mentioned previously can have a large effect on cine quality, the most significant gains are possible at the catheterization table. It is impressive how much difference there is between films taken by a careful angiographer who pays attention to the small details and those taken by one who rushes through without concern for the subtleties. In some cases, change of a centimeter or two in position can make the difference between proper exposure and underexposure (see Fig. 1-18).

Collimation and Shielding

Proper collimation of the x-ray beam serves two main purposes. First, by restricting the x-ray beam to the area of the intensifier that will be recorded on the cine film, unnecessary exposure to the patient is eliminated. Second, smaller x-ray fields result in less scatter radiation. Because scatter causes both image degradation and increased radiation dose to patient and personnel, this is also desirable. On the other hand, if the field is restricted too much, extensive panning is required, which adds motion unsharpness and can be very distracting. Radical collimation can result in overexposure of the film because part of the x-ray field is occupied by the lead collimator blades (Fig. 6-2).

Contour collimators, colloquially referred to as shields, are absolutely necessary for the performance of good angiography. To understand why, remember that the generator selects the x-ray parameters based on the average density within the circular area that occupies the central portion of the intensifier. If all of the density within this area is uniform, then the required exposure is also uniform, but if there are gross discrepancies in the various densities within the

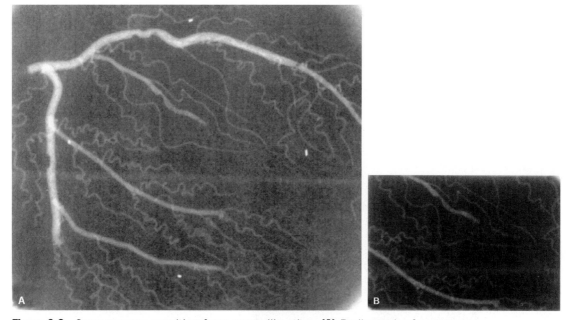

Figure 6-2. Overexposure resulting from overcollimation. **(A)** Radiograph of a coronary artery phantom with the collimators open is properly exposed. **(B)** With radical collimation, the automatic brightness control tries to penetrate the lead collimators, resulting in marked overexposure of the phantom.

sensing area, the calculated exposure will be a compromise. This may result in adequate exposure of one area and improper exposure of a second area, or improper exposure of the entire frame. By adding density to selected areas of lower density such as the lung, shields help create a more uniform x-ray field (Fig. 6-3A). This can be especially important along the anterior border of the heart in the cranial right anterior oblique view (Fig. 6-3B), where it is very easy to overexpose the LAD and diagonals as they course along the anterolateral wall.

Positioning and Panning

Proper positioning can make or break a cine run because it affects both film density and need for panning. When positioning the heart in the x-ray field, try to keep away from the edges of the intensifier because of distortion of the image caused by pincushion effect (see Fig. 5-7). Also,

depending on the framing, some of the image seen on video will not be on the cine film (see Fig. 1-5). Conversely, if the heart is too far away from the edges of the field, extra panning is required, with an attendant increase in motion unsharpness. It takes a fair amount of experience to be able to estimate how deeply the patient will breathe and compensate for that when initially positioning the patient under the intensifier. Once one can consistently do this, there will be no need to position with a deep breath. Paying attention to how deeply the patient inspires on the first cine runs will help in this regard.

Limited panning is one mark of a good angiographer. Few things are more distracting during interpretation of cineangiograms than constant and rapid panning. Panning can also be a source of significant motion unsharpness. The goal should be to use as little motion as possible and to pan in steps rather than continuously. Furthermore, there is rarely any reason to return to the starting point of the pan, especially with injection of the LIMA (Fig. 6-4). Some angiog-

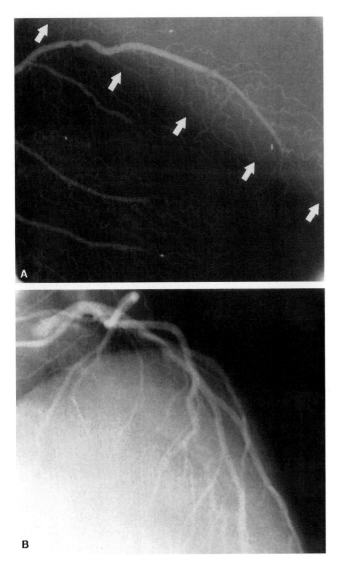

Figure 6-3. Countour collimators. **(A)** Straight contour collimator *(arrows)*. **(B)** Extreme cranial right anterior oblique view of the left coronary artery. A curved contour collimator (not readily apparent in this picture) has been positioned along the heart border, resulting in proper exposure of the left anterior descending, diagonals, and ramus intermedius, despite the presence of the diaphragm in the x-ray field.

raphers seem to use the "rub-a-dub-dub" method of panning, in which they make two or three complete circuits of the heart with each injection. It is important to resist the urge to constantly be panning.

There are other factors that affect the amount of panning necessary. Heart size is one factor about which not much can be done; however, minimization of overall magnification by keeping the intensifier close to the chest wall and using some judgment in choosing image intensifier mode allows more of the heart to be on the image and therefore decreases the amount of panning necessary. Use of total over-framing requires more panning because less

of the image area is used to expose the cine film (see Fig. 1-5).

In addition to overpanning, another habit to be avoided is rotating the x-ray gantry during filming. Although this may make for interesting pictures, it is a significant source of motion unsharpness: not only is there motion from the rotation, but all gantries vibrate to some degree, further exacerbating the problem.

Contrast Dose

The only reason the coronary arteries can be imaged radiographically is because of the iodine

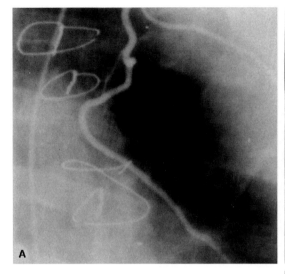

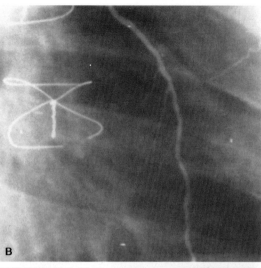

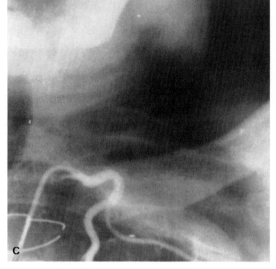

Figure 6-4. "Pandemonium" during filming of a left internal mammary artery (LIMA) graft to the left anterior descending. **(A–C)** The table is panned from the origin of the LIMA to the distal anastomosis and then, inexplicably, back past the origin of the LIMA.

that is added to the blood within them. If there is too little contrast material in a coronary artery, it will not be imaged adequately. There are two common causes of poor opacification: underfilling and low iodine content of the contrast material.

Underfilling of a coronary is all too common. The usual reason is underinjection secondary to what we facetiously refer to as "thenar palsy." This results in streaming of contrast material along the dependent wall of the vessel and may be difficult to recognize in any view other than a straight lateral view (Fig. 6-5). Some angiographers seem to have a pathologic fear of contrast material and do not give adequate injections

There are other causes, however. High coronary flow in conditions such as aortic stenosis, aortic regurgitation, hypertension, and dilated cardiomyopathy make it very difficult to opacify the coronary arteries because of dilutional effects. Sinus tachycardia may also contribute. This problem is compounded by the use of 5- and 6-Fr catheters. Strong consideration should be given to use of 7- or 8-Fr catheters with any condition that may cause either increased myocardial mass or high coronary flow.

The concentration of iodine in the contrast material is also important and can be decreased either by the manufacturer or by mixing of blood or saline with contrast material in the

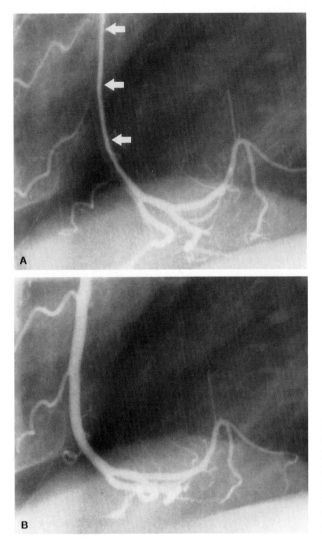

Figure 6-5. Lateral views of the right coronary artery demonstrating contrast streaming. **(A)** Inadequate injection rate early during the injection has resulted in the appearance of narrowing throughout the mid portion of the RCA. **(B)** After the force of injection is increased, the vessel fills completely and no narrowing is seen.

syringe. Any dilution of the contrast material adversely affects vessel opacification. Currently available contrast materials for cardiac angiography vary in iodine content from 320 to 370 mg/mL, an almost 14% difference. Although this difference may not be noticeable in thin patients, in whom the films are taken with low kVp, as the beam energy rises, the degradation in image quality becomes apparent (see Fig. 1-16). Because of this effect, it is the author's opinion that contrast material containing less than 350 mg of iodine per milliliter should not be used for coronary angiography.

QUALITY CONTROL

The final ingredient in the recipe for quality coronary angiograms is quality control: all the attention to angiographic technique and radiographic factors will be for naught if the films do not come out of the cine processor properly developed. It is beyond the scope of this text to go into the details of how to establish and maintain a quality control program, but a few important points should be made.

The most obvious area for quality control is the cine processor. Although they are in general

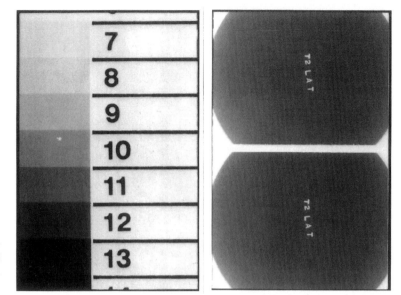

Figure 6-6. Quality control. Sensitometry strip *(left)* is used to check processor parameters. Density strip *(right)* checks for proper x-ray exposure.

quite reliable, processors have been known to underdevelop, overdevelop, and destroy cine film. Film destruction is obvious, but more subtle abnormalities can escape detection for long periods without regular testing and charting of processor parameters. This should be done on a daily basis and should include a density strip for each camera in each laboratory and a sensitometry strip for each processor (Fig. 6-6). The density strips should be made with a 1- to 2-mm copper plate on at least the most

commonly used image intensifier mode. The densities of several adjacent frames of each strip should be inspected for gross uniformity and then measured with a densitometer to obtain an average film density, which should be plotted on a chart on which the upper and lower limits of acceptable film density have been clearly marked (Fig. 6-7). The quality control person can then immediately determine whether the films will be of a satisfactory overall density. If the density of one or more of these strips is not within toler-

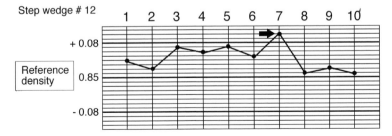

Figure 6-7. Daily density plot. Plotting the density measurements taken from the daily density strips allows one to readily identify when the density measurement is outside acceptable limits (in this case, ±0.08 density units) and any trends that may need correction before the density becomes too great or too little. In this case, density was on the high side of acceptable from days 3 through 6 and then exceeded limits on day 7 *(arrow)*. Corrective action at that time resulted in a return to ideal density.

ance, the sensitometry strip can be analyzed to determine whether the problem is in the x-ray equipment or the processor.

A sensitometry strip is made by exposing a strip of cine film in a sensitometer, a device that incorporates a constant light source with a step wedge. This produces a series of different densities on the sensitometry strip, which can then be measured with a densitometer and plotted to form a curve (Fig. 6-8) called an H & D curve, after Hurter and Driffield, who first published the technique in England in 1890. The H & D curve allows the laboratory personnel to determine film contrast and look for subtle aberrations in processor function. This is important both for immediate analysis of film problems and for long-term tracking of processor performance. If the sensitometry measurements are within tolerance, one can be fairly certain that the cause of abnormal film density is in the x-ray equipment. If not, then the processor problem must be corrected before the x-ray equipment can be evaluated.

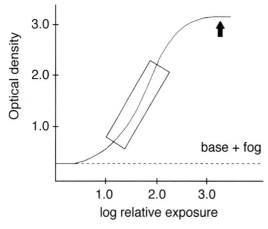

Figure 6-8. H & D curve. The logarithm of the relative exposure is plotted against optical density. Minimum film density *(dashed line)* is determined by film base plus any fog and should be as low as possible. Exposures at the upper end of the curve *(arrow)* result in film that is too dark and do not allow any further change in density with increasing exposure. The mid portion of the curve *(box)* provides a usable range of film density. The slope of the curve in this region is proportional to film contrast.

It does no good to perform daily quality control if the results are not analyzed before the performance of any cineangiography. Although it is most likely that everything will be satisfactory, films occasionally are lost because nobody was aware that the processor or x-ray equipment was malfunctioning. Unless the cineangiographer is willing to tell some patients that they need a second study because the films did not come out, it is suggested that a program of quality control be maintained with near-religious zeal.

You should feel free to call on your cine film company sales representative to educate your laboratory staff about how to perform quality control. It is in the company's best interest for your films to be as good as possible. Any company that does not provide this service should be replaced with one that will. In the final analysis, the service provided by the film manufacturer is far more important than the subtle differences between various brands of cine film. An all-too-common scenario is for the film quality in a laboratory that does not perform quality control to gradually drop over time to the point at which even an unobservant person can see that the films are not adequate. At that point, a new sales representative comes in and promises better results, which are easy to achieve by replacing the film and chemicals with their own and, more importantly, tuning up the processor, cleaning the cine camera, and performing overdue routine maintenance. The credit for improved images goes to the new film, when in fact the old film would have been perfectly satisfactory had the cine system been maintained. Unfortunately, if the laboratory reverts to its old ways and does not institute routine quality control, the new film will eventually look as bad as the old, and the cycle will begin anew.

SUMMARY

Coronary angiography demands more attention to detail than almost any other angiographic technique. The difference between a good film and an inadequate film may hinge on a few centimeters of positioning. Other than errors in positioning, there is no one factor that makes a tremendous difference, but the sum of errors resulting from careless angiographic technique can have a profound effect on study quality and hence patient benefit. Although it may take a few more minutes to properly set up positioning, collimation, shielding, and angiographic views, the benefits quickly become apparent and are worth the extra time and effort.

To summarize, to obtain optimum image quality, the cineangiographer should adhere to the following precepts:

1. As long as kVp can be kept below 90, use a small focal spot and a pulse width of less than 8 msec.

2. Use 30 frames per second for most applications.

3. Avoid high magnification (5-inch) intensifier mode.

4. Practice good positioning, collimation, and shielding.

5. Limit panning.

6. Give an adequate dose of contrast material.

7. Keep the image intensifier as close to the chest wall as possible.

8. Make certain that the x-ray equipment is functioning properly with daily quality control and routine maintenance.

With diligence, the pictures obtained can be the best possible for each patient with the available equipment.

BIBLIOGRAPHY

Culverwell RH. Radiographic imaging techniques for cardiology. In: Elliott LP. Cardiac imaging in infants, children and adults. Philadelphia: JB Lippincott, 1991:90.

Curry TS, Dowdey JE, Murry RC. Christensen's physics of diagnostic radiology. 4th ed. Philadelphia: Lea & Febiger, 1990.

Gray JE, Winkler NT, Stears J, Frank ED. Quality control in diagnostic imaging. Baltimore: University Park Press, 1983.

Levin DC, Dunham LR, Stueve R. Causes of cine image quality deterioration in cardiac catheterization laboratories. Am J Cardiol 1983;52:881.

*I*NDEX

Page numbers followed by f indicate figures; those followed by t indicate tabular material.